STUDENT WORKBOOK AND GUIDE FOR

CORE CONCEPTS IN PHARMACOLOGY

THIRD EDITION

LELAND NORMAN HOLLAND, JR., PhD

Hillsborough Community College, SouthShore Center

MICHAEL PATRICK ADAMS, PhD, RT(R)

Pasco-Hernando Community College

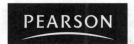

PEARSON

Boston   Columbus   Indianapolis   New York   San Francisco   Upper Saddle River
Amsterdam   Cape Town   Dubai   London   Madrid   Milan   Munich   Paris   Montreal   Toronto
Delhi   Mexico City   Sao Paulo   Sydney   Hong Kong   Seoul   Singapore   Taipei   Tokyo

Notice: Care has been taken to confirm the accuracy of information presented in this textbook. The authors, editors, and publisher, however, cannot accept responsibility for errors or omissions or for consequences from application of the information in this textbook and make no warranty, expressed or implied, with respect to its contents.

The authors and publisher have exerted every effort to ensure that drug selections and dosages set forth in this textbook are in accord with current recommendations and practices at the time of publication. However, in view of ongoing research, changes in government regulations, and the constant flow of information relating to drug therapy and drug reactions, the reader is urged to check the package inserts of all drugs for any change in indications of dosage and for added warnings and precautions. This is particularly important when the recommended agent is a new and/or infrequently employed drug.

Publisher: Julie Levin Alexander
Assistant to the Publisher: Regina Bruno
Editor-in-Chief: Maura Connor
Senior Acquisitions Editor: Kelly Trakalo
Editorial Assistant: Lauren Sweeney
Development Editor: Michael Giacobbe
Managing Production Editor: Patrick Walsh
Production Liaison: Yagnesh Jani
Production Editor: Mary Tindle, S4Carlisle Publishing Services
Manufacturing Manager: Ilene Sanford
Senior Art Director: Maria Guglielmo
Cover Designer: Wanda Espana
Director of Marketing: David Gesell
Marketing Coordinator: Michael Sirinides
Marketing Assistant: Crystal Gonzalez
Composition: S4Carlisle Publishing Services
Cover Printer: Lehigh Phoenix Color
Printer/Binder: Edwards Brothers Malloy
Cover Image: Courtesy of Maud S. Bech/Phototake, Inc.

Pearson Education LTD.
Pearson Education Singapore, Pte. Ltd
Pearson Education, Canada, Ltd
Pearson Education—Japan

Pearson Education Australia PTY, Limited
Pearson Education North Asia Ltd
Pearson Educación de Mexico, S.A. de C.V.
Pearson Education Malaysia, Pte. Ltd

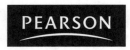

www.pearsonhighered.com

10 9 8 7 6 5 4
ISBN 13: 978-0-13-612109-1
ISBN 10: 0-13-612109-8

Contents

PREFACE

Students entering the field of nursing have a tremendous amount to learn in a very short time. This concise student workbook and resource guide has been developed to help you learn and apply key concepts and procedures and master critical-thinking skills based on *Core Concepts in Pharmacology*, 3e

At the beginning of each chapter you will find an Explore MyNursingKit box. Just as in the main textbook this box identifies some specific resources available at http://www.mynursingkit.com for the chapter. In addition, each chapter includes a variety of questions and activities to help you comprehend difficult concepts and reinforce basic knowledge gained from textbook reading assignments. Highlights of this workbook include:

- Chapters that correlate directly to *Core Concepts in Pharmacology*, 3e to allow you to easily locate information related to each question.
- Thorough assessment of essential information in the chapter through generous use of multiple-choice, fill-in, and matching style questions.
- Making Connections questions encourage you to recall concepts from previous chapters and apply them to the current chapter, thus promoting retention of information and continuity of learning.
- Dosage calculation problems provide additional practice to assist you in mastering this challenging topic.
- Clinical case studies provide in-depth scenarios to sharpen critical-thinking skills.
- Answers are included in an appendix to provide immediate reinforcement. It also allows you to check the accuracy of your work.

It is our hope that this workbook contributes to your success in beginning the study of the exciting and challenging subject of pharmacology.

CHAPTER 1

INTRODUCTION TO PHARMACOLOGY: DRUG REGULATION AND APPROVAL

LEARNING OUTCOMES

To view the objectives, please refer to the textbook or MyNursingKit™ at www.mynursingkit.com.

TRUE/FALSE

For Questions 1–8, choose T for true or F for false.

T F 1. Pharmacology is the science of pharmacy.

T F 2. An understanding of chemistry is not necessary for health care providers who educate and give advice to patients regarding their drug therapy.

T F 3. Biologics are drugs, naturally produced in animal cells, in microorganisms, or by the body.

T F 4. If prescription drugs have an exceptionally high margin of safety, regulators may change their status to over-the-counter (OTC) drugs.

T F 5. Throughout history, pharmaceutical ingredients have generally been regulated in the same manner as other drug products.

T F 6. Postmarketing surveillance rarely influences how long a drug will be marketed to consumers.

T F 7. The FDA Modernization Act of 1997 represents the largest reform effort of the drug review process since 1938.

T F 8. Drugs and the actions of health care professionals are the most powerful weapons we have against worldwide epidemics and diseases.

 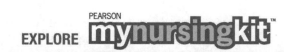

FILL IN THE BLANK

From the text, find the correct word(s) to complete the statement(s).

9. Chemical therapeutic agents that produce biological responses in the body are known as _____.

10. Herbs, extracts, vitamins, minerals, and dietary supplements are examples of _____ therapies.

11. Pharmacotherapy involves the science of _____ and _____.

12. The _____ was the first comprehensive publication established for standardization of drug purity, strength, and directions for synthesis in 1820. The second publication, called the _____, was originally drafted by the _____, founded in 1852.

13. In 1938, the _____ Act was the first legislation preventing the marketing of untested drugs.

14. The second stage of drug approval, called _____, takes place in three phases.

15. In Canada, the federal department responsible for health and safety regulation is _____.

16. Two things that are required before drugs in Canada can be sold are a _____ and _____, both assigned by Health Canada.

MATCHING

For Questions 17–20, match the stage of the U.S. drug approval process in Column I with its description in Column II.

Column I

17. _____ Stage I

18. _____ Stage II

19. _____ Stage III

20. _____ Stage IV

Column II

a. A new drug application (NDA) is reviewed while clinical Phase III trials continue. An NDA, if approved, grants exclusive rights to marketing for 17 years.

b. Postmarketing surveillance: Clinicians monitor the effects of the drug after it has been marketed.

c. Clinical investigation: Clinical pharmacologists perform studies in human subjects.

d. Preclinical investigation: Scientists perform experiments using animal and tissue culture models.

21. Place the six steps of the Canadian drug approval process in order.

_____ _____ _____ _____ _____ _____

a. Health Canada issues a Notice of Compliance (NOC) and Drug Identification Number (DIN), which permit the manufacturer to market the drug.

b. Health Canada monitors the effectiveness and concerns of the drug by regular inspection, notices, newsletters, and feedback from consumers and health care providers.

c. A drug company completes a drug submission to Health Canada that shows details of important safety and effectiveness information, including how the drug product will be produced and packaged, expected therapeutic benefits, and adverse reactions.

d. A committee of experts reviews the drug submission to identify potential benefits and drug risks.

e. Health Canada reviews information about the drug product and passes on important details to health care practitioners and consumers.

f. Preclinical studies or experiments involving tissue culture, living cells, and small animals are performed, followed by extensive clinical trials or testing done in humans.

MULTIPLE CHOICE

22. Which of the following statements best conveys the complicated nature of pharmacology?

a. There are over 10,000 brand and generic varieties of drugs with many different names, interactions, side effects, and complex mechanisms of action.

b. Many drugs may be prescribed for more than one disease and produce many different actions in the body.

c. Drugs may elicit different responses, depending on factors such as sex, age, health status, body mass, and genetics.

d. All of the above statements convey the complicated nature of pharmacology.

23. The branch of medicine dealing with the general treatment of suffering and disease is:

a. Pharmacotherapeutics

b. Pathophysiology

c. Therapeutics

d. Physiology

24. Which of the following choices distinguishes a traditional drug from a biologic or natural alternative agent? A traditional drug is:

a. Used routinely by health care practitioners

b. An extract from a natural source

c. Chemically produced

d. Associated with the bloodstream

25. Therapeutic drugs differ from foods, household products, and cosmetics in that:

a. Only therapeutic drugs can induce a biological response.

b. Foods, household products, and cosmetics are not traditionally designed for the treatment of disease and suffering.

c. Drugs may not be considered a part of the body's normal activities.

d. Drugs are narrowly defined.

26. Which of the following statements best describes an advantage of prescription drugs over OTC drugs?

a. OTC drugs do not require a physician's order.

b. Prescription drugs ensure that harmful reactions, ineffective treatment, or a progressive disease state will not occur.

c. Only patients authorized to receive prescription drugs will take these medications.

d. The practitioner can maximize therapy by ordering the amount and frequency to be dispensed.

27. Which branch of the Food and Drug Administration (FDA) handles approval of vaccines and hormones?

    a. Center for Drug Evaluation and Research (CDER)

    b. Center for Biologics Evaluation and Research (CBER)

    c. Center for Food Safety and Applied Nutrition (CFSAN)

    d. Center for Devices and Radiological Health

28. Clinical phase trials:

    a. Are extremely useful drug evaluations due to the potential variability of responses observed among patients

    b. Generally take less time than the preclinical investigation process

    c. Are a way to evaluate the effectiveness of a drug after it has been marketed to the general public

    d. Begin only after an NDA has been submitted to the FDA for approval

29. The FDA was officially established as an agency of the U.S. Department of Health and Human Services in:

    a. 1862

    b. 1906

    c. 1938

    d. 1988

30. In Canada, pharmaceutical drugs, including the narcotics, controlled and restricted drugs, and biologics, are specifically regulated by the:

    a. Therapeutic Products Programme (TPP)

    b. Office of Natural Health Products

    c. Food Directorate

    d. Health Protection Branch of the Department of Health and Welfare

31. Some consumers are concerned that the FDA Modernization Act of 1997 has:

    a. Enabled the FDA to collect too much money from drug and biologic manufacturers

    b. Allowed the FDA to hire too many employees

    c. Allowed drugs to be approved for therapeutic use in the United States at a faster rate than risks can be assessed

    d. Restructured its own organization in an adverse way

32. The devastation caused by bioterrorist activity or natural disasters would primarily be associated with which of the following factors?

    a. Little time to develop antidotes

    b. Inability to identify, isolate, and treat widespread diseases

    c. Widespread harm or illness, including panic and major casualties

    d. Overwhelming of health care services

CASE STUDY APPLICATIONS

33. Mr. A has a problem with mild constipation. This symptom has just occurred and does not seem to be related to a major illness. He has considered trying OTC drugs, such as Ex-Lax and Metamucil, but would like to know what natural alternative therapies he might consider.

    a. Given your knowledge of natural alternative therapies, what possible advantages might there be in Mr. A trying this approach rather than in considering OTC medication first?

    b. Would prescription drugs offer any advantage in this case?

34. Ms. B experiences what appears to be an unfavorable drug reaction and feels there is a problem with her medication. You are somewhat certain that the problem is not related to an inferior medical product, but to be extremely sure you cannot rule out this possibility.

    a. As a health professional, what kind of information could you give to Ms. B to help her understand the possible source of her problem?

    b. Should the manner in which patients report unfavorable reactions be different, depending on whether the type of drug therapy is prescription, OTC, or natural alternative?

35. During a routine visit to her doctor, Mrs. M confides to you that she is "terrified" of getting anthrax, even though no new cases have been reported in quite some time. She wants a supply of drugs to prevent an infection. You note that she becomes agitated while discussing terrorism, wringing her hands and looking distressed. Your nursing diagnosis is "Knowledge deficit related to bioterrorism/anthrax as evidenced by questions voiced and nonverbal anxiety behaviors."

    a. Your care plan includes interventions relating to patient education. What information would you give Mrs. M regarding prophylactic use of antibiotics for bioterrorism agents?

    b. What information would you give her about anthrax vaccine?

CHAPTER 2

DRUG CLASSES, SCHEDULES, AND CATEGORIES

LEARNING OUTCOMES

To view the objectives, please refer to the textbook or MyNursingKit™ at www.mynursingkit.com.

TRUE/FALSE

For Questions 1–7, choose T for true or F for false.

T   F   1. When drugs are grouped together on the basis of how they work pharmacologically, this is referred to as a therapeutic classification.

T   F   2. A prototype drug is the original, well-understood drug model from which other medications in a therapeutic class have been developed.

T   F   3. A drug's trade name, or proprietary name, is assigned by the company marketing the drug.

T   F   4. One of the main arguments against substituting generic drugs for brand name drugs is differences in bioavailability.

T   F   5. All scheduled drugs require a prescription in order to be dispensed.

T   F   6. The restrictions placed on controlled drugs are the same in the United States as they are in Canada.

T   F   7. Category X is the most harmful pregnancy drug category.

 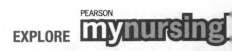

FILL IN THE BLANK

From the text, find the correct word(s) to complete the statement(s).

8. With _____ classifications, drugs are organized on the basis of their usefulness in treating a particular disorder.

9. Drugs organized by _____ classifications are categorized based on how they produce their effects in the body.

10. How a drug produces its effect in the body is referred to as its _____.

11. The description given to a drug by the International Union of Pure and Applied Chemistry (IUPAC) is its _____ name.

12. Drugs with more than one generic ingredient are called _____.

13. The overwhelming feeling that drives someone to use a drug repeatedly is known as _____.

14. _____ drugs are classified according to their potential for abuse.

15. In Canada, _____ drugs are medications used in the course of a chemical or an analytical procedure for medical, laboratory, industrial, educational, or research purposes.

MATCHING

For Questions 16–20, match the drug schedules in Column I with their descriptions in Column II.

Column I	**Column II**
16. _____ Schedule I	a. Used therapeutically without prescription
17. _____ Schedule II	b. High psychological/moderate physical dependency potential; dispensed with prescription
18. _____ Schedule III	
19. _____ Schedule IV	c. High abuse potential; dispensed with prescription
20. _____ Schedule V	d. Limited or no therapeutic use
	e. Low abuse potential; dispensed with prescription

For Questions 21–25, match the pregnancy categories in Column I with their descriptions in Column II.

Column I	**Column II**
21. _____ Category A	a. Studies have NOT shown a risk to women or to the fetus.
22. _____ Category B	b. Use of this drug MAY cause harm to the fetus, but it may provide benefit to the mother if a safer therapy is not available.
23. _____ Category C	
24. _____ Category D	c. Animal studies HAVE shown a risk to the fetus, but controlled studies have not been performed in women.
25. _____ Category X	
	d. Studies HAVE shown a significant risk to women and to the fetus.
	e. Animal studies have NOT shown a risk to the fetus or, if they have, studies in women have not confirmed this risk.

MULTIPLE CHOICE

26. Drugs are placed into therapeutic categories on the basis of:

    a. How the drug therapy is applied

    b. Mechanism of action of the drug

    c. Therapeutic usefulness of the drug

    d. Pharmacologic focus of the drug

27. The pharmacologic prototype approach to drug therapy considers the:

    a. Most popular drug for a particular disorder

    b. Most commonly used drug in a particular class

    c. Representative drug for how other drugs in a particular class work

    d. Drug of choice for a particular disorder

28. The preferred and less complicated drug name given by the United States Adopted Name Council is the:

    a. Generic name

    b. Brand name

    c. Chemical name

    d. Trade name

29. Generic drug names are preferred over other drug names for all of the following reasons EXCEPT:

    a. There may be dozens of product names for a particular drug.

    b. Chemical names are often complicated and difficult to remember or pronounce.

    c. Health care professionals most often use generic drug names when describing a medication.

    d. The generic drug name is an assigned name that can be consistently matched with a medication's active ingredients.

30. Drugs are sometimes placed on a negative formulary list because:

    a. Brand name drugs are generally more expensive than generic drugs.

    b. Many generic drugs have active ingredients that are more tightly compressed than those in brand name medications.

    c. Some generic drugs are unsafe to substitute for equivalent brand name products.

    d. Health care practitioners need to know which generic drug equivalents are considered unsafe.

31. In the United States, controlled substances are drugs:

    a. Whose use is restricted by the Controlled Substances Act of 1970 and later revisions

    b. Subject to guidelines outlined in Part III, Schedule G of the Food and Drugs Act

    c. Not intended for human use, covered in Part IV, Schedule H of the Food and Drugs Act

    d. Designated as Schedule F drugs, those requiring a prescription for their sale

32. A teratogen is:

    a. A substance having the potential to produce dependency

    b. Any substance that will harm a developing fetus or embryo

    c. A drug used exclusively for research purposes

    d. A drug whose use is restricted without a prescription

33. In Canada, drugs subject to guidelines outlined in Part III, Schedule G of the Food and Drugs Act should have which of the following labels on the outside of the medication vial?

    a. C

    b. F

    c. G

    d. N

34. According to the U.S. Drug Enforcement Agency (DEA), which of the following drug categories has the highest abuse potential?

    a. Schedule I

    b. Schedule II

    c. Schedule III

    d. Schedule IV

35. Which of the following drug categories is the safest in terms of its teratogenic effects?

    a. Category A

    b. Category B

    c. Category C

    d. Category D

CASE STUDY APPLICATIONS

36. Mrs. H, a prospective mother, will undoubtedly experience many uncomfortable symptoms during her pregnancy, including infections, skin rash, headaches, back pain, constipation, restlessness, difficulty sleeping, and a feeling of being extremely tired. There are many over-the-counter (OTC) and prescription medications normally used to treat many of these symptoms. Consider the following drug choices. Which would most likely be considered safe for Mrs. H? For those not recommended, give a rationale based on your knowledge of drug schedules and/or pregnancy categories. Use a drug guide to help with your answers.

    a. Penicillin V (Pen-Vee-K) for infection

    b. Acetaminophen (Tylenol) for headaches

    c. Naproxen (Anaprox, Naprosyn) for body aches and pains

    d. Castor oil (Purge) for constipation

    e. Diazepam (Valium) for difficulty sleeping

37. You are giving a hospitalized patient her morning medications. The patient asks you why you are giving the generic form acetaminophen instead of the trade product, Tylenol. The patient asks if there is a difference between trade and generic products.

    a. What is your best reply?

    b. The patient also asks if Tylenol is a controlled substance. What is your best reply?

CHAPTER 3

METHODS OF DRUG ADMINISTRATION

LEARNING OUTCOMES

To view the objectives, please refer to the textbook or
MyNursingKit™ at www.mynursingkit.com.

TRUE/FALSE

For Questions 1–8, choose T for true or F for false.

T   F   1. A drug administered by the enteral route is one given by
any route other than the digestive tract.

T   F   2. Drugs are introduced into the body during the
pharmacodynamic phase.

T   F   3. Of the three physical compositions of drugs, gaseous drugs generally produce the fastest onset
of action.

T   F   4. Sublingual and rectal administration routes are two examples in which drugs bypass destructive enzymes
of the liver.

T   F   5. Medications delivered by the oral route generally have a faster onset of action than those delivered
by the IM route.

T   F   6. The deepest type of injection made into the skin is called an intradermal injection.

T   F   7. Drugs applied to the nasal membranes, eyes, ears, or reproductive openings are considered to be topical
medications.

T   F   8. Transmucosal drugs are generally those delivered to the upper and lower respiratory tract
and reproductive openings.

 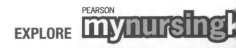

FILL IN THE BLANK

From the text, find the correct word(s) to complete the statement(s).

9. The _____ route means the nurse will administer the drug to the patient by mouth, under the tongue, or into the rectum.

10. When the nurse places a drug directly onto the skin or associated membranes, this is referred to as the _____ route.

11. The _____ phase of drug delivery involves four processes in the body: absorption, distribution, metabolism, and excretion.

12. _____ and _____ are two physical properties of a liquid drug that influence its movement throughout the body.

13. Drugs swallowed, chewed, or slowly dissolved in the mouth are referred to as _____ medications.

14. _____ administration involves placing drugs under the tongue.

15. _____ and _____ are examples of rectal administration methods.

16. The most common parenteral method of drug delivery is the _____ route.

17. Drugs are injected directly into the muscle in the _____ route.

18. A(n) _____ injection is made directly into the spinal subarachnoid space; a(n) _____ injection is made into the space overlying the dura mater.

19. One popular method for delivering drugs across the skin at a slow, steady rate is the _____ patch.

20. _____ drug delivery methods are useful in treating respiratory and reproductive ailments.

MATCHING

For Questions 21–31, match the specific drug delivery method in Column I with its general route in Column II.

Column I		Column II
21. _____ Rectal		a. Enteral
22. _____ Intravenous (IV)		b. Parenteral
23. _____ Intramuscular (IM)		c. Topical
24. _____ Oral (PO)		
25. _____ Transmucosal		
26. _____ Subcutaneous (SC or SQ)		
27. _____ Transdermal		
28. _____ Sublingual		
29. _____ Intrathecal (IT)		
30. _____ Intradermal		
31. _____ Subarachnoid		

For Questions 32–40, match the traditional drug formulation in Column I with its physical composition in Column II.

Column I	Column II
32. _____ Inhalants	a. Solids
33. _____ Suppositories	b. Liquids and liquid mixtures
34. _____ Lozenges	c. Gases
35. _____ Drops	
36. _____ Creams	
37. _____ Aerosols	
38. _____ Capsules	
39. _____ Ointments	
40. _____ Tablets	

MULTIPLE CHOICE

41. Which of the following statements about dissolution should the nurse consider correct?

    a. The shorter the dissolution time, the more delayed the onset of action.

    b. Water, taken in combination with solid drug formulations, is meant only to help dissolve the drugs.

    c. The process of dissolving solid drugs is dissolution.

    d. Dissolution time is only important for the drug administration phase of drug delivery.

42. After being administered, a medication must then be absorbed to produce an effect. After the medication is absorbed, which phase of drug delivery is occurring?

    a. Pharmaceutical phase

    b. Pharmacokinetic phase

    c. Pharmacodynamic phase

    d. None of the above

43. Of the following patients, which would be appropriate for rectal administration?

    a. Unconscious patient

    b. Patient experiencing nausea or vomiting

    c. Infant who cannot swallow pills

    d. All of the above

44. Which of the following drug delivery methods is NOT a parenteral method of drug delivery and avoids the first-pass effect in the liver?

    a. Oral

    b. Intrathecal

    c. Intramuscular

    d. Sublingual

45. Which of the following is a major advantage of IV drug administration?

    a. The duration of drug action can be easily controlled.

    b. It is relatively free from the possibility of harmful effects.

    c. A precise concentration of drug can be administered into the bloodstream.

    d. The onset of drug action can be easily controlled.

46. What is a disadvantage of subcutaneous drug delivery?

    a. The final drug concentration within the bloodstream is unpredictable.

    b. Drugs cannot be confined to a precise location.

    c. For safety reasons, patients must be conscious when they receive a subcutaneous injection.

    d. Pain, swelling, or infection may occur if proper precautions are not taken.

47. If rapid onset of action were critical, which of the following routes would the nurse choose?

    a. Intravenous

    b. Intramuscular

    c. Sublingual

    d. Rectal

48. Which of the following drug administration methods would the nurse use for the tuberculin test with purified protein derivative (PPD)?

    a. Topical

    b. Intradermal

    c. Subcutaneous

    d. Intramuscular

49. Implants are generally administered by which drug delivery method?

    a. Intradermal

    b. Subcutaneous

    c. Intraperitoneal

    d. Intramuscular

50. Which of the following drug delivery methods might be used when fast delivery to the cerebral spinal fluid is necessary?

    a. Intraperitoneal

    b. Intrathecal

    c. Epidural

    d. Transmucosal

51. Which of the following is true about the physical properties of drugs?

    a. Substances that are able to dissolve in lipids (fats) are called hydrophilic.

    b. Hydrophobic drugs mix well in the bloodstream but move less efficiently across body membranes.

    c. Drugs with lipid properties mix well with components of cellular membranes.

    d. All of the above are correct.

52. Which of the following statements is true about IV infusions?

    a. Single drug doses are generally administered over a shorter period.

    b. A flow regulator is always used to regulate drug flow.

    c. Quick delivery of IV drugs is not possible with IV infusion.

    d. Drug doses are generally administered by way of a syringe and needle.

53. What is the deepest skin layer?

    a. Epidermis

    b. Dermis

    c. Hypodermis

    d. Muscular layer

54. Which of the following statements is true regarding topical drug applications?

    a. For a local effect, it is necessary to keep drugs from penetrating the skin barrier.

    b. Liquids and liquid mixtures are the most effective physical compositions for topical drug therapy.

    c. In some cases, it is desirable for topical drugs to enter the systemic circulation.

    d. All of the above are correct.

55. What is the most common type of drug formulation for eye and ear medications?

    a. Salves

    b. Ointments

    c. Drops

    d. Sprays

CASE STUDY APPLICATIONS

56. In some cases, many different formulations are available, giving patients more than one option for drug therapy. Birth control is an example. Patients may take birth control pills, receive injections, or take medication via transdermal patches or vaginal inserts. Each method has advantages and disadvantages. Consider a situation in which your patient, a 34-year-old working mother, has an active lifestyle and needs a reliable and effective means of birth control.

    a. What assessment data should be gathered?

    b. Outline the patient teaching necessary to help this patient make the best choice.

57. An elderly man presents with a complaint of nausea and diarrhea. After a thorough assessment, the physician determines that medication might help relieve some of these symptoms and asks the nurse to administer the medication.

    a. In planning drug administration routes, what would you recommend for this patient and why?

    b. How will the nurse evaluate effectiveness of this route of administration?

CHAPTER 4

What Happens After a Drug Has Been Administered

LEARNING OUTCOMES

To view the objectives, please refer to the textbook or MyNursingKit™ at www.mynursingkit.com.

TRUE/FALSE

For Questions 1–10, choose T for true or F for false.

T F 1. Pharmacokinetics describes how drugs change body responses.

T F 2. Absorption is generally faster across thinner membranes compared with thicker membranes.

T F 3. Drugs that are more highly bound to plasma proteins are distributed more easily than drugs that are not bound to plasma proteins.

T F 4. Young and elderly patients usually metabolize drugs more slowly than middle-age patients.

T F 5. The main organs involved with excretion are the kidneys; however, other involved organs include the lungs, gallbladder, skin, and associated glands.

T F 6. A drug with a half-life of 5 hours will take longer to be eliminated from the body than a drug with a half-life of 10 hours.

T F 7. Factors influencing the success of drug therapy include drug dosing, frequency of dosing, and a changing medical condition.

T F 8. According to the receptor theory, most drug actions can be linked to a specific receptor.

T F 9. Drug antagonists are facilitators of drug action.

T F 10. The term *potency* refers to the ability of a drug to produce a more intense response as the concentration is increased.

 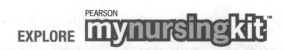

FILL IN THE BLANK

From the text, find the correct word(s) to complete the statement(s).

11. The four major areas of pharmacokinetics are _____, _____, _____, and _____.

12. The brain, placenta, and testes have barriers that prevent some drugs from gaining access through normal circulation. These are the _____ barrier, the _____ barrier, and the _____ barrier.

13. _____ is a process whereby most drugs are deactivated when passing through the liver.

14. Agents that become more active as they are exposed to detoxifying organs, such as the liver and kidneys, are called _____.

15. A mechanism called the _____ decreases the activity of most drugs traveling through the liver.

16. Breakdown products of drug metabolism are called _____.

17. Drugs secreted in the bile are often recycled in the liver because of a mechanism referred to as _____.

18. As discussed in the text, rate of elimination and _____ are two variables helpful in determining how long a drug will remain in the bloodstream and are thus indicators of how long drug action will last.

19. _____ deals with how drugs affect body responses.

20. The classic theory about the cellular mechanism by which most drugs produce a response is called the _____ theory.

21. _____ is a drug's strength at a particular concentration or dose, whereas _____ is the effectiveness of a drug in producing a more intense response as the concentration is increased.

MATCHING

For Questions 22–26, match the factors influencing drug effectiveness in Column I with the area of pharmacokinetics or pharmacodynamics in Column II.

Column I	Column II
22. _____ Concentration (dose) of an administered drug	a. Pharmacokinetics
23. _____ Presence of food in the digestive tract	b. Pharmacodynamics
24. _____ Frequency of drug dosing	
25. _____ Age of the patient	
26. _____ Kidney disease	

For Questions 27–35, match the factors affecting absorption in Column I with the absorption/ distribution rates shown in Column II.

Column I

27. _____ Warmer dispensing temperature

28. _____ Absence of food in the digestive tract

29. _____ Smaller surface area at the absorption site

30. _____ Binding of a drug to plasma proteins

31. _____ Thin membranes (as found in the lungs)

32. _____ Ability to mix with lipids

33. _____ Chemically charged (not neutral)

34. _____ Larger drug particle

35. _____ Thicker membranes (as found in the skin)

Column II

a. Faster absorption/distribution rate

b. Slower absorption/distribution rate

MULTIPLE CHOICE

36. The process of moving a drug from its site of administration across one or more body membranes is called:

   a. Absorption

   b. Distribution

   c. Metabolism

   d. Excretion

37. The process that describes how drugs are transported in the body is:

   a. Absorption

   b. Distribution

   c. Metabolism

   d. Excretion

38. The term used to describe how much of a drug is available to produce a biological response is:

   a. Volume of distribution

   b. Rate of elimination

   c. Bioavailability

   d. Half-life ($t_{1/2}$)

39. The fact that the half-life ($t_{1/2}$) of Drug A is longer than that of Drug B might be explained by a higher:

    a. Metabolic rate for Drug A

    b. Rate of elimination for Drug B

    c. Potency for Drug A

    d. Effectiveness for Drug B

40. One reason that the first-pass effect is so important is that drugs absorbed at the level of the digestive tract:

    a. Are circulated directly back to the heart

    b. Are distributed to the rest of the body and their target organs

    c. Have ultimately more bioavailability than they would if absorbed at a different location

    d. Are routed through the hepatic portal circulation

41. Drug doses are often _____ when administered to children or the elderly.

    a. Decreased to account for increased metabolism

    b. Increased to account for increased metabolism

    c. Decreased to account for decreased metabolism

    d. Increased to account for decreased metabolism

42. The removal of larger drug metabolites from the bloodstream to the urine is referred to as:

    a. Filtration

    b. Reabsorption

    c. Secretion

    d. Recirculation

43. Which of the following statements is NOT correct regarding excretion by the lungs?

    a. Factors that affect gas exchange influence the respiratory excretion rate.

    b. The greater the flow of blood into lung capillaries, the greater the respiratory excretion rate.

    c. Drugs easily converted to gases, such as ethanol, are especially suited for excretion by the respiratory system.

    d. The lungs excrete most drugs as products of metabolism.

44. For drugs easily dissolved in bile:

    a. Enterohepatic recirculation significantly decreases the duration of drug action.

    b. The entire drug amount is absorbed with the bile in the intestinal tract.

    c. Drugs are not subject to metabolism by the liver.

    d. A fraction of the drug amount is eliminated from the body through defecation.

45. Which of the following is most important regarding excretion mechanisms and the breasts?

    a. Drugs excreted into breast milk may significantly harm the nursing infant.

    b. The breasts are a modified type of sweat gland.

    c. Urea and other waste products are eliminated naturally from the breasts.

    d. Natural alternative agents are considered safe and are not excreted into breast milk.

46. Antagonists:

    a. Are sometimes referred to as facilitators of drug action

    b. Can produce an effect only by interacting with receptors

    c. Inhibit or block the action of agonist drugs

    d. Are all of the above

47. Consider a plot of where the Y-axis is labeled as percent of maximum response and the X-axis is labeled as time. If two S-shaped curves appear on the graph as identical except for their placement along the X-axis, the line on the left represents a drug that is:

    a. More potent

    b. Less potent

    c. Effective

    d. Less effective

48. If two S-shaped curves appear on a graph when one line is shorter and reaches a lower maximum response than the other line, the shorter line represents a drug that is:

    a. More potent

    b. Less potent

    c. More effective

    d. Less effective

49. For the figure below, which drug appears to be the most POTENT?

    a. X

    b. Y

    c. Neither; both have the same potency.

50. For the figure below, which drug appears to be the most EFFECTIVE?

    a. X

    b. Y

    c. Neither; both have the same effectiveness.

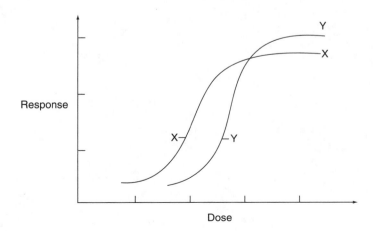

CASE STUDY APPLICATIONS

51. Mr. P is anxious and has not been able to sleep well for several weeks. He is moderately obese and has a history of hypertension and diabetes. After examination, the health care practitioner agrees to provide this patient with a drug to treat anxiety.

   a. What assessment data support the fact that drug distribution could be a problem for this patient?

   b. How will the nurse evaluate the effectiveness of the drugs used to treat anxiety?

   c. What is the primary site for excretion of this patient's medications and, therefore, the system that must be consistently evaluated by the nurse?

52. Mr. A is 60 years old and has been abusing alcohol for years. He appears to have no major medical problems. He has been admitted to an outpatient setting for a diagnostic evaluation of his bowel by colonoscopy.

   a. What elements of his history would alert the nurse to possible problems with pharmacokinetics?

   b. What interventions might the nurse expect during the medication phase of this procedure?

   c. What system(s) should the nurse assess following the delivery of any medications for this patient?

53. A patient with a history of severe migraines is taking an analgesic that is classified as an agonist/antagonist. The patient has not asked for the analgesic for 3 hours.

   a. What nursing assessment would you perform before giving this analgesic?

   b. What nursing diagnosis would you consider before giving this analgesic?

   c. What questions would you ask if the migraine headaches are not relieved within 15 minutes?

54. You are a nurse working with patients in an infectious disease clinic. Several of the patients are complaining that their wound infections are not healing quickly enough. You review their medical records.

   a. What information are you looking for related to pharmacotherapy?

   b. What outcomes would you expect to measure for the patient in a wound management clinic?

   c. What evaluation would support your recommendation for a medication change?

CHAPTER 5

PHARMACOLOGY AND THE NURSING PROCESS

LEARNING OUTCOMES

To view the objectives, please refer to the textbook or MyNursingKit™ at www.mynursingkit.com.

TRUE/FALSE

For Questions 1–5, choose T for true or F for false.

T F 1. It is not necessary that an initial patient assessment include herbs and dietary supplements taken by the patient because these have no impact on drug therapy outcomes.

T F 2. Specific actions that the nurse should take to move the patient toward a stated health goal are called assessments.

T F 3. When evaluating the outcomes of pharmacotherapy the nurse should always assume that the patient has taken the drug as directed.

T F 4. The first step in the planning phase is for the nurse to identify the desired goal or outcome.

T F 5. A nurse who is comparing baseline assessment data to current objective data is performing the evaluation phase of the nursing process.

FILL IN THE BLANK

From the textbook, find the correct word(s) to complete the statement(s).

6. _____ data are what the patient says or perceives, such as pain, anxiety, or nausea.

7. Conditions that have caused or contributed to the patient's problems are called _____.

8. A primary nursing role is to enable patients to become _____ _____ in their own care.

 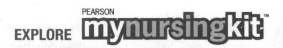

9. The _____ _____ is a systematic method of problem solving that forms the foundation for nursing practice.

10. A _____ _____ is a clinical judgment of an actual or potential health problem of the patient that is within the nurse's scope of practice to address.

11. Taking a prescribed drug incorrectly, or not taking the drug at all, is called _____.

MATCHING

For Questions 12–18, match the description in Column I with the nursing process step in Column II.

Column I	Column II
12. _____ First step in the nursing process	a. Evaluation
13. _____ Data that include what the patient says	b. Intervention
14. _____ Data gathered through diagnostic sources	c. Nursing diagnoses
15. _____ Provide the basis for planning patient care	d. Objective data
16. _____ Objective measure of goals	e. Subjective data
17. _____ Links strategies to established outcomes	f. Assessment
18. _____ Assessment of goals and outcomes	g. Outcomes
	h. Planning

MULTIPLE CHOICE

19. Mr. J has just returned from surgery. As the nurse, you are taking vital signs, checking his incision site, and determining if he is in pain. With these actions, what step of the nursing process are you using?

    a. Evaluation

    b. Planning

    c. Assessment

    d. Intervention

20. Mr. J has begun to complain of pain in his incision site. As the nurse, you are to administer morphine sulfate 2 mg IV. With these actions, what step of the nursing process are you using?

    a. Evaluation

    b. Planning

    c. Assessment

    d. Intervention

21. Mr. J has inquired about the physical therapy he will be receiving to regain his mobility after his knee replacement surgery. As the nurse, you will interact with physical therapy to coordinate his plan of care. With these actions, what step of the nursing process are you using?

    a. Evaluation

    b. Planning

    c. Assessment

    d. Intervention

22. Mr. J received the physical therapy and has regained his mobility after his knee replacement surgery. As the nurse, you interact with physical therapy to determine if he is ready to be discharged from the skilled unit. With these actions, what step of the nursing process are you using?

    a. Evaluation

    b. Planning

    c. Assessment

    d. Intervention

23. Ms. L is complaining of pain in her right hip and a burning sensation in the area around her incision. As the nurse, you are recording these findings. What type of information have you gathered?

    a. Objective data

    b. Subjective data

    c. Outcomes

    d. Goals

24. Ms. L is complaining of pain in her right hip. As the nurse, you have assessed the area and have found swelling, redness, and open areas, and there is a history of trauma to the hip. What type of information have you gathered?

    a. Objective data

    b. Subjective data

    c. Outcomes

    d. Goals

25. Ms. L is complaining of pain in her right hip. As the nurse, you have assessed the area and have found swelling, redness, and open areas, and there is a history of trauma to the hip. This information may be used to compare with assessment information gathered at a later date. What type of information have you gathered?

    a. Objective data

    b. Subjective data

    c. Outcomes

    d. Baseline data

26. Mrs. C is recovering from a fracture of the right hip. The interdisciplinary team has established a schedule of physical therapy for her. She will ambulate using a walker with the assist of one member of the team for 50 feet three times a day for 1 week, to be increased to 100 feet three times a day for 2 weeks, then to be changed to a quad cane and standby assist for 2 weeks and then discharged to home. What type of information has been presented?

    a. Outcomes

    b. Goals

    c. Baseline data

    d. Objective data

27. What factor established from the patient's health history would suggest the greatest potential for nonadherence to the medication regimen?

    a. Male

    b. Female

    c. Elderly

    d. Lives in a rural area

28. The nurse is developing goals and outcomes for Ms. D who is being discharged today following recent abdominal surgery. One key element regarding these goals is that they:

    a. Should be patient oriented

    b. Should be nurse oriented

    c. Should include at least three outcomes

    d. Should not be seen by the patient prior to discharge

29. The nurse writes "Mobility, Physically Impaired" on a patient's record. This statement is considered a/an:

    a. Intervention

    b. Outcome

    c. Nursing diagnosis

    d. Assessment

DO YOU REMEMBER?

30. All drugs have more than one:

    a. Name

    b. Active ingredient

    c. Generic name

    d. Indication

31. How do therapeutic drugs differ from foods, household products, and cosmetics?

    a. Only therapeutic drugs can induce a biologic response.

    b. Food, household products, and cosmetics are not traditionally designed for the treatment of disease and suffering.

    c. Drugs may not be considered part of the body's normal activities.

    d. Drugs are narrowly defined.

32. Which method is used for delivering large volumes of medications?

    a. Intradermal

    b. Intravenous

    c. Intramuscular

    d. Subcutaneous

33. To produce an effect, most drugs must interact or bind to:

    a. Another drug

    b. Plasma proteins

    c. A specific receptor

    d. Hepatic enzymes

34. What is the process of moving a drug from its site of administration across one or more body membranes to circulating fluids called?

    a. Absorption

    b. Metabolism

    c. Distribution

    d. Excretion

CASE STUDY APPLICATIONS

35. Ms. P is 15-year-old teenager who has just been diagnosed with type 1 diabetes mellitus. She has presented to the emergency department on three occasions with blood glucose of over 400. She is grossly obese and has not been compliant in following her prescribed diet and insulin regimen.

    a. What would be some potential nursing diagnoses for this patient?

    b. What goals would you establish for improving adherence to the medication regimen?

36. Mrs. G is a 35-year-old Hispanic migrant worker who does not speak or understand English. She presents to the emergency department with severe abdominal pain and rigidity in the right lower quadrant. As the nurse in charge, you are to take the health history and establish a plan of care. What barriers would you expect to encounter when establishing her plan of care, and how might they be overcome?

37. Mr. W is a 25-year-old patient with a history of substance abuse. He has been admitted to your area after receiving critical injuries in a car wreck. He is now recovering and has moved to the acute ward from intensive care unit (ICU). As the nurse establishing his plan of care, what goals and outcomes will you establish for this patient?

CHAPTER 6

HERBS AND DIETARY SUPPLEMENTS

LEARNING OUTCOMES

To view the objectives, please refer to the textbook or MyNursingKit™ at www.mynursingkit.com.

TRUE/FALSE

For Questions 1–4, choose T for true or F for false.

T F 1. Because they are natural substances, herbal products have no adverse effects on the body.

T F 2. The Dietary Supplement Health and Education Act of 1994 (DSHEA) requires that herbal products be tested for effectiveness before they may be marketed.

T F 3. Most complementary and alternative medicine (CAM) therapies have been subjected to rigorous scientific studies that have compared their effectiveness with that of prescription drugs.

T F 4. An herb is technically defined as the woody tissue of a plant, such as the stems or bark.

FILL IN THE BLANK

From the text, find the correct word(s) to complete the statement(s).

5. Herbal products are regulated by the _____ Act.

6. From the perspective of pharmacology, the value of CAM therapies lies in their ability to _____ the need for _____.

7. Ginger should be used cautiously, if at all, in patients with _____ disorders.

 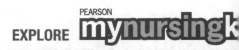

MATCHING

For Questions 8–12, match the description in Column I with the herb or dietary supplement in Column II.

Column I	Column II
8. _____ Antitoxin, protection against liver disease	a. Valerian
9. _____ May reduce depression	b. St. John's wort
10. _____ Relieves stress and promotes sleep	c. Cranberry
11. _____ Prevents urinary tract infection	d. Milk thistle
12. _____ Heals skin scrapes or burns	e. Aloe

MULTIPLE CHOICE

13. With the rising of the pharmaceutical industry in the late 1800s, interest in herbal medicine began to wane because:

    a. Herbs became very expensive.

    b. Herbs were no longer readily available in the environment.

    c. Synthetic drugs could be standardized and produced more cheaply.

    d. Herbs were proven to be ineffective against most diseases.

14. Which of the following is NOT a major factor contributing to the recent increase in popularity of botanicals?

    a. Many herbs have been clearly demonstrated to be more effective than available drugs.

    b. Herbal products are more widely available to the public.

    c. The herbal industry has aggressively marketed its products.

    d. Herbal products cost considerably less than most prescription medicines.

15. Products intended to enhance the diet, such as botanicals, vitamins, minerals, or any other extract or metabolite that is not already approved as a drug by the Food and Drug Administration (FDA), are defined as:

    a. Herbal products

    b. Alternative therapies

    c. Supplemental therapies

    d. Dietary supplements

16. Which of the following is a legal requirement contained in the DSHEA?

    a. Dietary supplements must be tested for safety prior to marketing.

    b. Effectiveness must be demonstrated by the manufacturer.

    c. The herbal product must contain only one active ingredient.

    d. Dietary supplements must state that the product is not intended to diagnose, treat, cure, or prevent any disease.

17. Which of the following statements would most likely NOT be allowed on the label of a dietary supplement?

    a. Helps promote a healthy immune system

    b. May reduce pain and inflammation

    c. Reduces blood pressure and the risk for stroke

    d. May improve cardiovascular function

18. Which popular herb is used for its possible benefit in treating depression?

    a. Aloe

    b. Soy

    c. St. John's wort

    d. Ginger

19. Which popular herb is used for its possible beneficial effect on the immune system?

    a. Black cohosh

    b. Echinacea

    c. Gingko

    d. Valerian

20. The nurse/health professional would be most likely to recommend saw palmetto for which of the following?

    a. Relief of urinary problems related to prostate enlargement

    b. Reduction of stress and promotion of sleep

    c. Reduction of blood cholesterol levels

    d. Treatment of constipation

21. Many patients use _____ to relieve premenopausal and menopausal symptoms.

    a. Milk thistle

    b. Valerian

    c. Garlic

    d. Black cohosh

22. Patients taking anticoagulants should be advised not to take which herb?

    a. Echinacea

    b. Ginger

    c. Saw palmetto

    d. Garlic

23. The health care provider should advise patients NOT to take valerian if they:

    a. Are taking central nervous system (CNS) depressants

    b. Have a bleeding disorder

    c. Are taking insulin

    d. Have Parkinson's disease

CASE STUDY APPLICATIONS

24. Mr. K, a 42-year-old teacher, has been taking gingko biloba for 5 years since he was diagnosed with a memory disorder, yet he feels that his condition is worsening. He has also been taking echinacea regularly, yet he now has the flu and probably pneumonia. He is angry and feels that the advertisements in nutrition magazines and on television may have misled him into buying useless products. He is seeking advice from you regarding the value of alternative therapies.

   a. Modern research on alternative therapies may fail to demonstrate the positive benefits that have been reported in the historical and cultural record. Does this mean that these products are truly ineffective? How can you explain this to Mr. K?

   b. Can you think of some reasons that scientists have difficulty demonstrating the effects of botanicals?

25. Mrs. R comes to your mental health outpatient clinic with new symptoms, including agitation, headache, and dizziness. You note on assessment that she is also profusely diaphoretic. Mrs. R has been treated for depression with Prozac, a selective serotonin reuptake inhibitor (SSRI). During your assessment, she confides that she has been using St. John's wort with her prescription drugs. She asks if her prescription can be changed to something that "works better."

   a. What is a likely cause of Mrs. R's symptoms?

   b. Your initial plan of care is for patient education regarding drug-herb interactions. What other antidepressants might interact unfavorably with St. John's wort?

CHAPTER 7

SUBSTANCE ABUSE

LEARNING OUTCOMES

To view the objectives, please refer to the textbook or MyNursingKit™ at www.mynursingkit.com.

TRUE/FALSE

For Questions 1–10, choose T for true or F for false.

T F 1. The most commonly abused drugs are illegal substances.

T F 2. Several drugs once used for therapeutic purposes are now considered illegal.

T F 3. *Physical dependence* refers to an altered physical condition caused by the nervous system adapting to repeated drug use.

T F 4. Once a patient becomes psychologically dependent and the substance is discontinued, classic withdrawal symptoms occur.

T F 5. Immunity is a condition in which progressively higher doses of the drug are required in order to produce the same effect.

T F 6. The most common method by which nicotine enters the body is through the inhalation of cigarette, pipe, or cigar smoke.

T F 7. Marijuana smoke does not produce a significantly higher risk for lung cancer than cigarette smoke.

T F 8. Drug effects from hallucinogens are highly variable and dependent on the mood and expectations of the user and the surrounding environment in which the drug is used.

T F 9. Amphetamines, cocaine, methylphenidate, and caffeine are examples of misused central nervous system (CNS) stimulants.

T F 10. Most abused CNS depressants are either controlled or illegal.

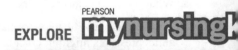

EXPLORE PEARSON mynursingk

www.mynursingkit.com

MyNursingKit is your one stop for online chapter review materials and resources. Prepare for success with additional NCLEX®-style practice questions, interactive assignments and activities, web links, animations and videos, and more! Register your access code from the front of your book at www.mynursingkit.com.

FILL IN THE BLANK

From the text, find the correct word(s) to complete the statement(s).

11. The most commonly abused drugs are _____ and _____.

12. Three substances that come from natural sources and are frequently abused are _____, _____, and _____.

13. The risk of addiction to prescription drugs is based on _____ and _____.

14. Two categories used to classify substance dependence are _____ and _____.

15. _____ occurs when a person has an overwhelming desire to take a drug and cannot stop.

16. Psychological dependence may develop after one dose of _____.

17. It is common to treat alcohol withdrawal with a short-acting _____.

18. Opioid withdrawal can be treated with _____.

19. After several months of pain therapy, a patient must increase the dose of the pain medication. The best description of this situation is that the patient has developed _____ for the pain medication.

20. All hallucinogenic drugs are Schedule _____ drugs.

21. _____ is a drug often applied via transdermal patch to ease signs of drug discontinuation, including agitation, weight gain, anxiety, headache, and an extreme craving.

22. Signs of physical discomfort after drug use is discontinued are referred to as classic _____ symptoms.

MATCHING

For Questions 23–30, match the drug or substance in Column I with its group name in Column II.

Column I	Column II
23. _____ Lysergic acid diethylamide (LSD)	a. Hallucinogen
24. _____ Pentobarbital (Nembutal)	b. CNS stimulant
25. _____ Alprazolam (Xanax)	c. CNS depressant
26. _____ Methadone (Dolophine)	d. Opioid
27. _____ Dextroamphetamine (Dexedrine)	
28. _____ Methylphenidate (Ritalin)	
29. _____ Propoxyphene (Darvon)	
30. _____ MDMA (Ecstasy)	

For Questions 31–35, match the symptoms of withdrawal in Column I with their drug classification in Column II.

Column I	**Column II**
31. _____ Depression	a. Opioid
32. _____ Dilated pupils	b. Nicotine
33. _____ Goose bumps	c. Cocaine
34. _____ Increased appetite	
35. _____ Yawning	

For Questions 36–39, match the drug/substance in Column I with its source in Column II.

Column I	**Column II**
36. _____ Opium	a. Natural
37. _____ MDMA	b. Synthetic
38. _____ Cocaine	
39. _____ LSD	

MULTIPLE CHOICE

40. All abused substances affect which body system?

    a. Cardiovascular

    b. Nervous

    c. Digestive

    d. Respiratory

41. You are working with a patient who has a diagnosis of alcoholism. What organ system is most likely to be malfunctioning for this patient?

    a. Lungs

    b. Bowels

    c. Liver

    d. Kidneys

42. A patient is admitted with liver failure. What nursing action is most appropriate prior to delivery of medications for this patient?

    a. Check drug dosing because of issues related to metabolism.

    b. Request increase in blood clotting drugs because of liver dysfunction.

    c. Hold all nutritional supplements until liver disease is resolved.

    d. Expect an increase in drug dosing of antibiotics because of immune compromise.

43. Repeated use of caffeine products can create which of the following effects?

    a. Decreased stomach acid

    b. Decreased blood pressure

    c. Increased fatigue

    d. Increased urination

44. What drug was once used for bronchodilation but has been discontinued because of psychotic episodes in some patients?

    a. Cocaine

    b. Lysergic acid diethylamide (LSD)

    c. Phencyclidine

    d. Amphetamine

45. Which of the following statements about addiction is NOT correct?

    a. Addiction is most likely a neurobiological problem linked closely to the patient's psychological state and social setting.

    b. In some cases, addiction may begin with the patient's medical need for the treatment of an illness.

    c. The therapeutic use of narcotics and sedatives creates large numbers of addicted patients.

    d. Attempts to predict a patient's addictive tendency using psychological profiles or genetic markers has largely been unsuccessful.

46. Which of the following drugs was once used as a local anesthetic?

    a. Amphetamine

    b. Ketamine

    c. Phencyclidine

    d. Cocaine

47. What is the condition in which a person has an overwhelming desire to take a drug and cannot stop?

    a. Addiction

    b. Dependence

    c. Tolerance

    d. Withdrawal

48. The situation in which an individual adapts to a drug over a short time and requires higher and higher doses to produce the same effect is called:

    a. Conditioning

    b. Withdrawal

    c. Immunity

    d. Tolerance

49. What is the sleep disorder drug class for which patients often fake or change prescriptions?

    a. Amphetamines

    b. Barbiturates

    c. Benzodiazepines

    d. Opioids

CASE STUDY APPLICATIONS

50. A 28-year-old patient is admitted to the hospital with pneumonia. During your assessment of the social history, you learn that the patient has a job, is self-reliant, and smokes marijuana every other night but does not drink alcohol. The patient claims, "Smoking a joint now and then doesn't hurt anybody."

    a. Based on your understanding of marijuana, what would you teach this patient regarding its long-term effects?

    b. Describe the psychological effects of marijuana and explain how dependence might develop in this case.

    c. Compare the marijuana risks with those of smoking tobacco products.

51. A patient admitted for recurrent bladder infections describes a 15-year history of drinking beer and wine in moderate amounts. The patient gives a family history of paternal alcoholism. The patient asks, "What kinds of factors are linked with addiction? Is it genetic, or is there some other reason people become addicted?"

    a. What would you include in the teaching plan to answer the patient's questions?

    b. What assessment data are important when you admit this patient?

    c. What nursing diagnoses and what patient outcomes would you write?

CHAPTER 8

DRUGS AFFECTING FUNCTIONS OF THE AUTONOMIC NERVOUS SYSTEM

LEARNING OUTCOMES

To view the objectives, please refer to the textbook or MyNursingKit™ at www.mynursingkit.com.

TRUE/FALSE

For Questions 1–10, choose T for true or F for false.

T F 1. Nerves from the autonomic nervous system provide voluntary control over skeletal muscle.

T F 2. The parasympathetic nervous system is activated under nonstressful conditions and produces symptoms associated with rest and digestion.

T F 3. When neurons are connected to each other at a synapse, the neurotransmitter is released from the postsynaptic nerve.

T F 4. Norepinephrine is the sympathetic neurotransmitter responsible for activating sweat glands.

T F 5. Acetylcholine stimulates receptors located within autonomic ganglia and organs associated with the parasympathetic nervous system.

T F 6. Norepinephrine receptors are of two basic subtypes, alpha (α) and beta (β).

T F 7. Cholinergic blockers produce symptoms associated with rest and digest.

T F 8. A sympathomimetic is a drug that inhibits the sympathetic nervous system.

T F 9. Parasympathomimetic drugs produce the same effects as activation of the parasympathetic nervous system.

T F 10. Two major categories of cholinergic receptors are muscarinic and nicotinic receptors.

 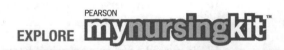

FILL IN THE BLANK

From the text, find the correct word(s) to complete the statement(s).

11. The two primary divisions of the nervous system are the _____ nervous system, made up of the brain and spinal cord, and the _____ nervous system.

12. The _____ nervous system provides involuntary control over smooth muscle, cardiac muscle, and glands.

13. The sympathetic nervous system produces the _____ response; the parasympathetic nervous system produces symptoms called the _____ response.

14. According to the textbook, three parts of a synapse are the _____ nerve, the _____, and the _____ nerve.

15. _____ is the main neurotransmitter responsible for sympathetic nervous transmission; _____ is the main neurotransmitter responsible for parasympathetic nervous transmission.

16. Sympathetic nerves are often called _____, which is from the word *adrenaline;* parasympathetic nerves are called _____.

17. Increased heart rate, bronchodilation, decreased motility in the gastrointestinal (GI) tract, mydriasis, and decreased secretions from glands are physiologic responses associated with inactivation of the _____ nervous system or activation of the _____ nervous system.

18. _____ blockers, primarily used for hypertension, comprise the most commonly prescribed autonomic medications.

19. A class of drugs named after the fight-or-flight response and primarily used for increasing the heart rate, dilating the bronchi, and drying secretions resulting from colds is _____ drugs.

20. _____ drugs, named after the rest-and-digest response, are commonly used to stimulate the urinary or digestive tract following general anesthesia.

MATCHING

For Questions 21–25, match the physiologic responses in Column I with the autonomic receptor classes in Column II.

Column I	Column II
21. _____ Cause dry mouth, constipation, urinary retention, and increased heart rate	a. Beta$_2$-drugs
	b. Alpha$_1$-blockers
22. _____ Relax vascular smooth muscle and dry nasal secretions	c. Beta$_1$-drugs
23. _____ Cause bronchodilation	d. Alpha$_1$-drugs
24. _____ Lower blood pressure without affecting the heart	e. Cholinergic (muscarinic) blockers
25. _____ Decrease heart rate	

For Questions 26–30, match the peripheral nervous system drug in Column I with the indication in Column II.

Column I	Column II
26. _____ Atropine (Isopto Atropine)	a. Myasthenia gravis
27. _____ Bethanechol (Urecholine)	b. GI stimulation following surgery
28. _____ Pyridostigmine (Mestinon)	c. Pupil dilation during an eye exam
29. _____ Doxazosin (Cardura)	d. Asthma inhaler
30. _____ Albuterol (Proventil)	e. Hypertension

For Questions 31–35, match the drug in Column I with the classification in Column II.

Column I	Column II
31. _____ Scopolamine (Hyoscine)	a. Parasympathomimetic
32. _____ Phenylephrine (Neo-Synephrine)	b. Anticholinergic
	c. Sympathomimetic
33. _____ Bethanechol (Urecholine)	d. Adrenergic blocker
34. _____ Propranolol (Inderal)	
35. _____ Dobutamine (Dobutrex)	

MULTIPLE CHOICE

36. A patient is discharged with a newly prescribed blocker for control of hypertension. The nurse gives discharge instructions. It is inappropriate to include which of the following instructions prior to the patient's leaving?

   a. Report any difficulty with urination.

   b. Take the medication for the first time directly prior to getting into bed.

   c. Monitor blood pressure (BP) and pulse daily.

   d. Return for laboratory tests to monitor renal function.

37. An adrenergic blocker is MOST DIRECTLY related to which of the following?

   a. Stimulation of the sympathetic nervous system

   b. Inhibition of the parasympathetic nervous system

   c. Stimulation of the parasympathetic nervous system

   d. Inhibition of the sympathetic nervous system

38. How does bethanechol (Urecholine) exert its effects?

   a. Stimulates cholinergic receptors

   b. Blocks cholinergic receptors

   c. Blocks beta receptors

   d. Stimulates alpha receptors

39. What drugs block the action of norepinephrine at alpha and beta receptors?

    a. Parasympathomimetics

    b. Parasympatholytics

    c. Sympathomimetics

    d. Sympatholytics

40. A nurse is to give phenylephrine parenterally. What safety precaution would be necessary especially with this drug?

    a. Monitor patency throughout the infusion.

    b. Monitor the temperature of the patient every 1 hour during the infusion.

    c. Monitor for central nervous system (CNS) depression.

    d. Monitor for hypotension throughout the infusion.

41. Parasympathomimetics are safe for patients diagnosed with which of the following?

    a. Myasthenia gravis

    b. GI obstruction

    c. Asthma

    d. Angina or dysrhythmias

42. How does propranolol (Inderal) exert its effects?

    a. Stimulates cholinergic receptors

    b. Blocks cholinergic receptors

    c. Blocks beta receptors

    d. Stimulates alpha receptors

43. Pseudoephedrine has been ordered for a patient with nasal congestion. The nurse knows that the drug can give which of the following side effects?

    a. Hypertension, insomnia, and tachycardia

    b. Drowsiness and dry mouth

    c. Increased heart rate and abdominal cramps

    d. Dilated pupils and orthostatic hypotension

44. Anticholinergics may be used in the treatment of peptic ulcers. What action makes this drug useful in this condition?

    a. Decreases gastric emptying time

    b. Decreases gastric acid secretions

    c. Decreases intestinal motility

    d. Relaxes gastric smooth muscles

45. What are sympathomimetics also called?

    a. Cholinergic drugs

    b. Adrenergic drugs

    c. Cholinergic blockers

    d. Adrenergic blockers

46. Epinephrine is a nonselective adrenergic drug. What is the disadvantage of this nonspecific action?

    a. It causes more autonomic side effects.

    b. This drug cannot be used for nervous system conditions.

    c. It will not cross the blood-brain barrier.

    d. It can be given only by subcutaneous injection.

47. A patient is prescribed Mestinon for myasthenia gravis. Which of the following would be inappropriate to teach the patient?

    a. Take the drug at the same times each day.

    b. Take the drug on a full stomach.

    c. Monitor liver enzymes as requested.

    d. Maintain a journal of episodes of weakness and how long they occur after the drug is given.

48. Neostigmine is an example of which of the following?

    a. Cholinergic blocker

    b. Nicotinic blocker

    c. Cholinergic drug

    d. Cholinesterase inhibitor

49. Which of the following drugs dry up body secretions?

    a. Bethanechol (Urecholine)

    b. Metoprolol (Lopressor)

    c. Atropine (Isopto Atropine)

    d. Doxazosin (Cardura)

50. Atropine is usually not prescribed for any patient with glaucoma. The nurse knows that the contraindication is due to which of the following effects of atropine?

    a. Increase in intraocular pressure

    b. Decrease in lacrimation

    c. Decrease in lateral movement of the eyes

    d. Increase in difficulty with night vision due to pupillary constriction

DO YOU REMEMBER?

51. Methylphenidate (Ritalin) is most similar to which abused substance?

    a. Tetrahydrocannabinol (THC)

    b. Ketamine

    c. Methamphetamine

    d. Ethyl alcohol

52. When a drug is referred to as an agonist, it can do which of the following?

    a. Be a facilitator of an action

    b. Be an inhibitor of an action

    c. Have a potentiated action

    d. Make one drug interact with another drug

53. What are the most commonly abused sympathomimetics?

    a. Amphetamines

    b. Proventil

    c. Sudafed/pseudoephedrine

    d. Marijuana

54. What is an example of an illegal CNS stimulant?

    a. Propoxyphene (Darvon)

    b. Flurazepam (Dalmane)

    c. Heroin

    d. Cocaine

55. The nurse is to administer medications using the "five rights." To give medications to a patient without an identification (ID) bracelet violates which of the rights?

    a. Right medications

    b. Right time

    c. Right patient

    d. Right route

CASE STUDY APPLICATIONS

56. Mr. Z, age 80, has been diagnosed with chronic obstructive pulmonary disease (COPD) and hypertension. The patient has been given propranolol (Inderal) to treat the hypertension. The nurse is assessing the following medications that he is also taking.

    Benadryl 25 mg every 4 hours for itching and sneezing due to allergies
    Prazosin bid for hypertension
    Proventil inhaler prn for wheezing

    a. Identify three potential nursing diagnoses that could occur due to drug interactions when these medications are given concurrently. Explain why these interactions could occur.

    b. What nursing interventions can be done to decrease the risk of the problems created with these interactions?

57. Ms. W, diagnosed with myasthenia gravis, comes to the emergency department (ED) with muscle weakness. During the history, the nurse determines that the patient has been taking double doses of her pyridostigmine (Mestinon) over the past several days.

    a. What assessment would the nurse make to identify a nursing diagnosis?

    b. What nursing diagnosis would you identify?

    c. What nursing interventions could be used in the diagnosis?

CHAPTER 9

DRUGS FOR ANXIETY AND INSOMNIA

LEARNING OUTCOMES

To view the objectives, please refer to the textbook or MyNursingKit™ at www.mynursingkit.com.

TRUE/FALSE

For Questions 1–8, choose T for true or F for false.

T F 1. Drug therapy for phobias, obsessive-compulsive disorders, and post-traumatic stress disorders (PTSDs) involves administration of anxiolytic drugs.

T F 2. The only major indication for benzodiazepine therapy is anxiety.

T F 3. The reasons for insomnia should be investigated thoroughly before considering drugs as a routine course of therapy.

T F 4. Benzodiazepines, barbiturates, and nonbarbiturates are classified as central nervous system (CNS) depressants.

T F 5. Patients should not expect to see adverse effects after discontinuing insomnia drugs abruptly.

T F 6. The electroencephalogram (EEG) is a tool that is sometimes used for diagnosing insomnia.

T F 7. Stages of non-REM and REM sleep are relatively unaffected by most sedative and sedative-hypnotic drugs.

T F 8. Although alcohol should be avoided with barbiturate and nonbarbiturate CNS depressants, it may be safely consumed with benzodiazepines.

 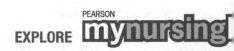

FILL IN THE BLANK

From the text, find the correct word(s) to complete the statement(s).

9. Apprehension, tension, or uneasiness lasting for 6 months or longer and causing considerable stress is referred to as _____.

10. Two important sets of brain structures are associated with anxiety. One connected with emotion is the _____ system; the other, projecting from the brainstem and connected with alertness, is the _____ system.

11. _____ are classes of drugs prescribed to relax patients. Classes of drugs used to help patients to sleep are _____.

12. Diazepam (Valium) reduces anxiety by binding to a receptor in the brain referred to as the _____ channel molecule.

13. The drug class usually prescribed for short-term insomnia caused by anxiety is _____.

14. _____ are a class of drugs that reduces anxiety, causes drowsiness, and promotes sleep when administered at higher doses.

15. _____ is a fatal symptom often associated with an overdose of barbiturates or other CNS depressants.

16. Schedule _____ is the level assigned to many benzodiazepines; Schedule _____ is the level assigned to some barbiturates.

17. _____ is a form of depression associated with reduced release of melatonin.

18. Non-REM and REM sleep are most affected by _____ drugs.

MATCHING

For Questions 19–23, match each description in Column I with its drug classification in Column II.

Column I	Column II
19. _____ Beginning in the early 1900s, the drug classification that has been used to control seizures, insomnia, and anxiety	a. Benzodiazepines
	b. Barbiturates
20. _____ Class containing drugs that act by binding GABA, intensifying the effect, without causing respiratory depression unless taken with other CNS depressants	c. Nonbenzodiazepines, nonbarbiturate sedatives
	d. Antidepressants
21. _____ Class containing older drugs rarely prescribed due to safer drugs, commonly prescribed for anxiety and insomnia	
22. _____ Class containing antihistamines, used in over-the-counter (OTC) sleep aids that do not cause dependency	
23. _____ Class containing drugs used for treating anxiety, phobias, and more serious mood-related disorders	

For Questions 24–29, match the drug in Column I with its class name and most appropriate use in Column II.

Column I	Column II
24. _____ Secobarbital (Seconal)	a. Benzodiazepine for anxiety and panic
25. _____ Chlordiazepoxide (Librium)	b. Benzodiazepine for short-term relief of insomnia
26. _____ Zolpidem (Ambien)	c. Barbiturate for short-term relief of insomnia
27. _____ Prazepam (Centrax)	d. Barbiturate for short-term sedation
28. _____ Amobarbital (Amytal)	e. Nonbarbiturate CNS depressant for short-term relief of insomnia
29. _____ Triazolam (Halcion)	

MULTIPLE CHOICE

30. What term describes episodes of immediate and intense apprehension, fearfulness, or terror?

   a. Anxiety

   b. Panic

   c. Phobia

   d. Post-traumatic stress

31. What drugs are meant to address anxiety on a more limited basis?

   a. Anxiolytics

   b. Sedatives

   c. Mood disorder drugs

   d. Antidepressants

32. Of the following, which is an inappropriate use of benzodiazepines?

   a. Long-term administration to treat phobias, obsessive-compulsive disorder (OCD), and PTSD

   b. Treatment of anxiety that interferes with daily activities of living

   c. Short-term treatment of generalized anxiety disorder

   d. Short-term treatment of insomnia caused by anxiety

33. Which of the following categorizes benzodiazepines?

   a. Sedative

   b. Hypnotic

   c. Tranquilizer

   d. All of the above

34. One of the first drugs used for anxiety treatment was:

   a. Alprazolam (Xanax)

   b. Clonazepam (Klonopin)

   c. Chlordiazepoxide (Librium)

   d. Clorazepate (Tranxene)

35. CNS depressants include which of the following drug classes?

    a. Benzodiazepines

    b. Barbiturates

    c. Nonbarbiturates, nonbenzodiazepine sedatives

    d. All of the above

36. Which statement is true about reestablishing a healthful sleep regimen?

    a. Drinking alcohol close to bedtime helps one to sleep.

    b. Eating a moderate meal close to bedtime helps one to sleep.

    c. Supplements are often recommended for insomnia.

    d. Sedatives and hypnotics may be useful for insomnia if taken long term.

37. Which of the following best describes rebound insomnia?

    a. It is a time during which insomnia and symptoms of anxiety may worsen.

    b. It is a worsening of insomnia due to drug dependency.

    c. It is more common in younger patients.

    d. It develops from short-term use of insomnia medication.

38. Melatonin can be bought over the counter for insomnia. Which patient teaching would be appropriate?

    a. Melatonin can increase ovulation in women who are trying to conceive.

    b. Melatonin can be taken safely during pregnancy.

    c. Melatonin can safely be given to patients who are on steroids.

    d. Melatonin is not regulated by the Food and Drug Administration (FDA), but it is sold over the counter without a prescription.

39. Which of the following is true regarding sleep stages and patterns?

    a. Drugs for insomnia generally do not affect sleep stages.

    b. Patients with normal sleep patterns move from non-REM to REM sleep about every 90 minutes.

    c. REM sleep is the deepest stage of sleep.

    d. The most significant type of sleep with respect to the effect of hypnotic drugs is REM sleep.

40. Sleep deprivation has been linked to which of the following?

    a. Decreased risk of type 2 diabetes

    b. Fear, irritability, paranoia, and emotional disturbance

    c. Less daydreaming or fantasizing throughout the day

    d. Better judgment and less impulsive thinking

41. Which of the following best describes phenobarbital?

    a. It is a short-acting barbiturate and thus more useful for brief medical procedures.

    b. It stimulates liver enzymes and thus may increase its own metabolism with repeated dosing.

    c. It is mainly limited in drug therapy for induction of sleep.

    d. It does not affect levels of folate (B_9) or vitamin D in the body.

42. Benzodiazepines must be given with caution when given parenterally due to what risk?

    a. Seizures

    b. CNS excitation

    c. Respiratory depression

    d. Dependence

43. Which of the following best describes buspirone (BuSpar)?

    a. It is a benzodiazepine.

    b. It may act by binding to brain dopamine and serotonin receptors.

    c. It is used for short-term treatment of insomnia.

    d. All of the above are correct.

DO YOU REMEMBER?

44. A patient is experiencing extreme anxiety in a dental chair due to an impending tooth extraction. Which route should the dentist use to give the most rapid onset of action?

    a. Oral

    b. IV

    c. IM

    d. Rectal

45. Scopolamine (Transderm-Scop) is an anticholinergic drug. Which of the following is LEAST likely to be a side effect of this drug?

    a. Dry mouth

    b. Bradycardia

    c. Tachycardia

    d. Urinary retention

46. Which of the following drug delivery methods is NOT a parenteral method of drug delivery and avoids the first-pass effect in the liver?

    a. Oral

    b. Epidural

    c. Intramuscular

    d. Sublingual

47. One reason that the first-pass effect is so important is that drugs absorbed at the level of the digestive tract:

    a. Are circulated directly back to the heart

    b. Are distributed to the rest of the body and target organs

    c. Have ultimately more bioavailability than they would if absorbed at a different location

    d. Are routed through the hepatic portal circulation

48. Younger and elderly patients metabolize drugs _____ middle-age patients.

    a. More slowly than

    b. More rapidly than

    c. At the same rate as

CASE STUDY APPLICATIONS

49. Mr. L is a 38-year-old patient who is to have a short surgical procedure during which he will be given Versed IV. The nurse knows that Versed is a short-acting benzodiazepine.

    a. What does the nurse need to assess prior to giving Versed?

    b. What interventions would the nurse use to maintain the patient's safety during the procedure?

    c. What would the nurse use to evaluate the effectiveness of these interventions?

50. Mrs. D has not slept well in weeks. She is troubled about a new job and feels that, if she can just get through a couple more weeks, things might start to become a little easier. One thing that would help Mrs. D is a good night's sleep.

    a. What nursing diagnosis would you identify for this patient?

    b. What nursing interventions would you use to assist this patient?

    c. What would you teach the patient regarding the pharmacologic interventions available?

CHAPTER 10

DRUGS FOR EMOTIONAL AND MOOD DISORDERS

LEARNING OUTCOMES

To view the objectives, please refer to the textbook or MyNursingKit™ at www.mynursingkit.com.

TRUE/FALSE

For Questions 1–9, choose T for true or F for false.

T   F   1.   Attention deficit disorder (ADD) is four to eight times more likely to occur in boys.

T   F   2.   Monoamine oxidase inhibitors (MAOIs) are drugs of choice for the treatment of simple depression.

T   F   3.   Tricyclic antidepressants (TCAs) produce fewer cardiovascular side effects and, therefore, are less dangerous than MAOIs.

T   F   4.   Patients taking lithium (Eskalith) should be placed on a salt-free diet to increase the effectiveness of the drug.

T   F   5.   Patients with psychosis are usually able to function normally in society without long-term medication.

T   F   6.   Many patients suffering from schizophrenia have family members who have experienced the same disorder.

T   F   7.   Atypical antipsychotic medications are effective for both positive and negative symptoms of psychosis.

T   F   8.   The inability to focus on a task or to pay attention is one of the main symptoms of ADD.

T   F   9.   A family history of depression raises the risk for a patient to experience biological depression.

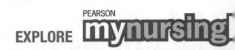

EXPLORE PEARSON mynursing

www.mynursingkit.com

MyNursingKit is your one stop for online chapter review materials and resources. Prepare for success with additional NCLEX®-style practice questions, interactive assignments and activities, web links, animations and videos, and more! Register your access code from the front of your book at www.mynursingkit.com.

FILL IN THE BLANK

From the text, find the correct word(s) to complete the statement(s).

10. Another name for mood disorders is _____ disorders.

11. The two major types of mood disorders are _____ and _____.

12. The three major classes of antidepressants are _____, _____, and _____.

13. _____ are drugs of choice for simple depression.

14. _____ produce fewer cardiovascular side effects and, therefore, are less dangerous than the MAOIs.

15. Patients taking _____ for bipolar disorder should be placed on a low-sodium diet to increase its effectiveness.

16. The inability to focus or pay attention is one of the main symptoms of _____.

17. _____ are the class of drugs most widely prescribed for ADD.

18. _____ disorder is depression associated with reduced release of melatonin during winter months.

19. Drugs for bipolar disorders are called _____ because they have the ability to modulate extreme shifts in emotions between _____ and _____.

MATCHING

For Questions 20–31, match the drug in Column I with its primary indication or class in Column II.

Column I	Column II
20. _____ Lithium carbonate (Eskalith)	a. ADD/CNS stimulant
21. _____ Venlafaxine (Effexor)	b. Depression/tricyclic type
22. _____ Paroxetine (Paxil)	c. Depression/MAOI
23. _____ Amitriptyline hydrochloride (Elavil)	d. Depression/SSRI
24. _____ Phenelzine sulfate (Nardil)	e. Depression/atypical or other
25. _____ Methylphenidate hydrochloride (Ritalin)	f. Bipolar disorder
26. _____ Pemoline (Cylert)	
27. _____ Tranylcypromine sulfate (Parnate)	
28. _____ Nortriptyline hydrochloride (Aventyl, Pamelor)	
29. _____ Bupropion hydrochloride (Wellbutrin)	
30. _____ Fluoxetine hydrochloride (Prozac)	
31. _____ Sertraline hydrochloride (Zoloft)	

For Questions 32–36, match the definition in Column I with its correct term in Column II.

Column I		Column II
32. _____	Enzyme that breaks down catecholamine neurotransmitters in the synapse	a. Amphetamines
33. _____	Accumulation of serotonin when taking two drugs that reduce serotonin uptake	b. Bipolar disorder
34. _____	Condition exhibiting signs of both clinical depression and mania	c. Monoamine oxidase
35. _____	Class of drug that is closely related to methylphenidate	d. Tyramine
36. _____	Chemical found in medications that cannot be ingested by patients on MAOIs due to high risk of severe hypertension	e. Serotonin syndrome

MULTIPLE CHOICE

37. What is the most common age range for the diagnosis of ADD?

    a. 0 to 3 years

    b. 3 to 7 years

    c. 10 to 13 years

    d. 15 to 18 years

38. Which medication has NOT been useful in stabilizing emotions in mood disorders such as bipolar disorder?

    a. Lithium (Eskalith)

    b. Carbamazepine (Tegretol)

    c. Valproic acid (Depakene)

    d. Pemoline (Cylert)

39. Lithium is used with other medications during phases of bipolar disorder. Which of these medications would NOT be used with lithium?

    a. Tricyclic antidepressants

    b. Benzodiazepines

    c. SSRI antidepressants

    d. Diuretics

40. Which of the following is an advantage of using Scattera instead of a scheduled CNS stimulant?

    a. Scattera improves the ability to focus and decreases hyperactivity.

    b. Scattera has shown more effectiveness than Ritalin.

    c. Scattera has fewer CNS side effects than Ritalin.

    d. Scattera is not as addictive as Ritalin.

41. A patient is sent home after being given fluoxetine (Prozac) for depression. The nurse should instruct the patient to do which of the following?

    a. Call back if there is no improvement in 24 hours.

    b. Call back if any nausea, drowsiness, or dizziness occurs.

    c. Start the Prozac before stopping the patient's present MAOI.

    d. Expect to see improvement in mood, appetite, and energy within 1 to 3 weeks.

42. Methylphenidate (Ritalin) produces its effects by activating what portion of the brain?

    a. Cerebellum

    b. Hypothalamus

    c. Pituitary

    d. Reticular activating system

43. When sending a patient home on imipramine (Tofranil), which of the following is important for the nurse to teach patients?

    a. St. John's wort may be used concurrently with no anticipated interaction.

    b. Photosensitivy is not a problem with Tofranil.

    c. This drug should not be stopped abruptly.

    d. Use of this drug with other CNS depressants is permitted.

44. Which of the following is NOT a common symptom of clinical depression?

    a. Lack of energy

    b. Sleep disturbances

    c. Hallucinations

    d. Feelings of despair or guilt

45. In assessing a patient, the nurse should know that rapid shifts in emotions from profound depression to euphoria and hyperactivity are characteristic of which of the following?

    a. Psychosis

    b. Bipolar disorder

    c. Schizophrenia

    d. ADD

46. Which of the following would LEAST likely be used to treat clinical depression?

    a. MAOIs

    b. Tricyclic antidepressants

    c. Selective serotonin reuptake inhibitors

    d. Phenothiazines

47. How does phenelzine (Nardil) produce its therapeutic effects?

    a. Inhibits the reuptake of norepinephrine into presynaptic nerve terminals

    b. Irreversibly inhibits MAO and intensifies the effects of norepinephrine in the synapse

    c. Selectively inhibits the reuptake of serotonin into presynaptic nerve terminals

    d. Interferes with the binding of dopamine to receptors located in the limbic system

48. How do tricyclic antidepressants produce their therapeutic effects?

    a. Inhibit the reuptake of both serotonin and norepinephrine into presynaptic nerve terminals

    b. Irreversibly inhibit MAO and intensify the effects of norepinephrine in the synapse

    c. Selectively inhibit the reuptake of serotonin into presynaptic nerve terminals

    d. Interfere with the binding of dopamine to receptors located in the limbic system

49. How does fluoxetine (Prozac) produce its therapeutic effects?

    a. Inhibits the reuptake of both serotonin and norepinephrine into presynaptic nerve terminals

    b. Irreversibly inhibits MAO and intensifies the effects of norepinephrine in the synapse

    c. Selectively inhibits the reuptake of serotonin into presynaptic nerve terminals

    d. Interferes with the binding of dopamine to receptors located in the limbic system

50. Why are the selective serotonin reuptake inhibitors (SSRIs) generally preferred over other classes of antidepressants?

    a. They are more effective.

    b. They produce fewer sympathomimetic and anticholinergic side effects.

    c. They do not produce sexual dysfunction.

    d. They cause more extrapyramidal effects.

51. The nurse should teach patients taking fluoxetine to avoid foods high in which amino acid because it is a chemical precursor for serotonin synthesis?

    a. Histidine

    b. Tyramine

    c. Lysine

    d. Tryptophan

DO YOU REMEMBER?

52. Typical oral doses are 1 mg for risperidone and 50 mg for clozapine. Which of the following may you correctly conclude from this information?

    a. Risperidone is more effective.

    b. Clozapine is more effective.

    c. Risperidone is more potent.

    d. Clozapine is more potent.

53. Thorazine is available by both IM and oral routes. Which would be expected to have a faster onset of action?

   a. IM

   b. Oral

54. In assessing a new patient, the nurse should know that panic attacks, phobias, and obsessive-compulsive disorders are usually treated with:

   a. Antipsychotic drugs

   b. Antianxiety drugs

   c. Drugs for bipolar disorder

   d. Antidepressants

55. "Speedball" is the street name for a drug combination containing methylphenidate (Ritalin) and which of the following?

   a. Heroin

   b. Marijuana

   c. LSD

   d. Cocaine

56. Methylphenidate is a Schedule II drug. What does this mean?

   a. It may adversely affect the fetus.

   b. It has no therapeutic use.

   c. It has a low abuse potential.

   d. It has a high potential for physical and psychological dependence.

CASE STUDY APPLICATIONS

57. A patient who has bipolar disorder has been started on lithium. He is also on paroxetine (Paxil), digoxin (Lanoxin), furosemide (Lasix), and potassium supplements for depression, hypertension, and congestive heart failure (CHF). He has also been on a low-sodium diet.

   a. During the first 3 weeks on lithium, what would the nurse identify as the priority nursing diagnosis?

   b. What assessments would the nurse make in identifying this diagnosis?

   c. What is the patient goal for the first 3 weeks of therapy?

58. A patient, Mrs. C, has been started on sertraline (Zoloft) for depression. On being admitted, she has been assessed as having episodes of crying, feelings of guilt, insomnia, and suicidal ideation. The nurse needs to monitor the patient for effectiveness, side effects, and potential problems. What goals might be assigned to the patient and how might those goals be evaluated?

CHAPTER 11

DRUGS FOR PSYCHOSES

LEARNING OUTCOMES

To view the objectives, please refer to the textbook or MyNursingKit™ at www.mynursingkit.com.

TRUE/FALSE

For Questions 1–5, choose T for true or F for false.

T   F   1. The vast majority of psychoses have no identifiable cause.

T   F   2. The most common psychiatric disorder characterized by abnormal thoughts, disordered communication, withdrawal, and suicidal risk is schizoaffective disorder.

T   F   3. The phenothiazines block dopamine D_2 receptors.

T   F   4. Atypical antipsychotic drugs treat both positive and negative signs of schizophrenia and have become drugs of choice for treating psychoses.

T   F   5. Drugs for psychoses have relatively few anticholinergic adverse effects.

 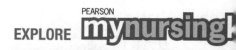

FILL IN THE BLANK

From the text, find the correct word(s) to complete the statement(s).

6. The most common type of psychosis is _____.

7. Psychoses may be classified as _____ or _____.

8. Chronic psychoses develop over _____, whereas acute psychoses develop in _____.

9. Atypical antipsychotic drugs are effective for both _____ and _____ symptoms of psychosis.

10. The majority of psychoses have no known _____. The six identifiable causes are _____, _____, _____, _____, _____, and _____.

11. Positive symptoms include _____, _____, _____, and _____.

12. Negative symptoms include a lack of _____, _____, _____, and _____.

13. Proper diagnosis of positive and negative symptoms is important for selection of the appropriate _____ drugs.

14. Symptoms of schizophrenia are thought to be associated with the _____ receptors in the basal nuclei.

15. Medications that block 65% of D_2 receptors will reduce symptoms of _____. Blocking more than 80% will likely cause _____ symptoms.

MATCHING

For Questions 16–25, match the drug in Column I with its primary indication or class in Column II.

Column I	Column II
16. _____ Haloperidol (Haldol)	a. Psychosis/phenothiazine
17. _____ Thioridazine (Mellaril)	b. Psychosis/nonphenothiazine
18. _____ Chlorpromazine (Thorazine)	c. Psychosis/atypical
19. _____ Prochlorperazine (Compazine)	d. Dopamine system stabilizer
20. _____ Olanzapine (Zyprexa)	
21. _____ Loxapine (Loxitane)	
22. _____ Clozapine (Clozaril)	
23. _____ Aripiprazole (Abilify)	
24. _____ Thiothixene (Navane)	
25. _____ Risperidone (Risperdal)	

For Questions 26–34, match the characteristic in Column I with its term and condition in Column II.

Column I

26. _____ A condition in which the patient exhibits symptoms of both schizophrenia and mood disorders

27. _____ Firm ideas and beliefs not founded in reality

28. _____ Symptoms that are added to normal behavior

29. _____ Antipsychotic medication

30. _____ An extreme suspicion that one is being followed or that others are trying to harm one

31. _____ Symptoms that subtract from a normal behavior

32. _____ False perceptions having no relation to reality

33. _____ A class of drug that might be used to decrease extrapyramidal effects

34. _____ A movement disorder brought on by medication effects

Column II

a. Paranoia

b. Delusions

c. Hallucinations

d. Positive symptoms

e. Negative symptoms

f. Schizoaffective disorder

g. Neuroleptic

h. Anticholinergics

i. Extrapyramidal effects

MULTIPLE CHOICE

35. Which class of drugs tends to produce severe side effects, such as muscle twitching, compulsive motor activity, and a Parkinson-like syndrome?

    a. Barbiturates

    b. Phenothiazines

    c. Benzodiazepines

    d. Serotonin reuptake inhibitors

36. Delusions, hallucinations, disordered communication, and difficulty relating to others are symptoms closely associated with which of the following?

    a. Clinical depression

    b. Bipolar disorder

    c. Schizophrenia

    d. ADD

37. Extrapyramidal side effects consist of:

    a. Paranoid delusions

    b. Profound depression

    c. Seizures

    d. Distorted body movements and muscle spasms

38. Like many antipsychotics, chlorpromazine (Thorazine) usually takes how long before its therapeutic effect is achieved?

    a. 2 to 3 days

    b. 2 to 3 weeks

    c. 7 to 8 weeks

    d. More than 6 months

39. Many of the major effects of chlorpromazine (Thorazine) can be attributed to which of the following?

    a. Inhibiting the reuptake of both serotonin and norepinephrine into presynaptic nerve terminals

    b. Irreversibly inhibiting monoamine oxidase (MAO) and intensifying the effects of norepinephrine in the synapse

    c. Selectively inhibiting the reuptake of serotonin into presynaptic nerve terminals

    d. Interfering with the binding of dopamine to receptors located throughout the brain

40. Why are atypical antipsychotics sometimes preferred over phenothiazines?

    a. They produce no major adverse effects.

    b. They can treat both positive and negative symptoms of psychosis.

    c. They are much more effective.

    d. They can improve symptoms within a few days of initial administration.

41. Nonphenothiazine agents differ from phenothiazine agents in what way?

    a. Nonphenothiazines do not produce as many anticholinergic side effects as phenothiazines.

    b. Nonphenothiazines cause less sedation and fewer anticholinergic side effects than phenothiazines.

    c. Phenothiazines do not produce as many side effects as nonphenothiazines.

    d. Phenothiazines cause less sedation and fewer anticholinergic side effects than nonphenothiazines.

42. Patients on clozapine (Clozaril) must watch carefully for signs of agranulocytosis, which include:

    a. Dizziness and drowsiness

    b. Appetite increase

    c. Fever and sore throat

    d. Bruises and bleeding

43. A patient who is on a phenothiazine complains of having elevated temperature, sweating, and "not feeling well." For what possible indication should the nurse assess the patient?

    a. Agranulocytosis

    b. Neuroleptic malignant syndrome

    c. Infection that may decrease potency of the medication

    d. Dystonic reaction

44. For a patient who has problems with daily compliance, a drug is available that lasts for 3 weeks. Which drug would be a good choice for this patient?

    a. Haloperidol (Haldol LA)

    b. Olanzapine (Zyprexa)

    c. Chlorpromazine (Thorazine)

    d. Clozapine (Clozaril)

45. A patient develops EPS after taking phenothiazines. The nurse would expect an order for which medication to counteract the EPS?

    a. Diphenhydramine (Benadryl)

    b. Procyclidine (Kemadrin)

    c. Levodopa (Larodopa)

    d. Tacrine (Cognex)

46. When a patient takes phenothiazines for an extended time, what conditions would the nurse expect to see?

    a. Parkinsonism

    b. Hypertensive crisis

    c. Decreased muscle rigidity

    d. Bruising and bleeding from the gums

DO YOU REMEMBER?

47. A patient has been prescribed an antipsychotic drug that has a high degree of anticholinergic side effects. Anticholinergic effects include which of the following?

    a. Nervousness and tremors

    b. Restlessness and constant movement of the legs

    c. Drying of the mouth, sedation, and urinary retention

    d. Headaches, skin rashes, and hallucinations

48. The atypical antipsychotics bind to serotonergic and cholinergic sites throughout the brain. The nurse understands that this would affect which neurotransmitters?

    a. Acetylcholine and serotonin

    b. Serotonin and dopamine

    c. Serotonin and norepinephrine

    d. Acetylcholine and norepinephrine

49. Benzodiazepines are often given with antipsychotic drugs. Which benzodiazepine side effects would create a problem when given with this class of antipsychotic medications?

    a. Drowsiness and dry mouth

    b. Lowered seizure threshold

    c. Hypotension and respiratory depression

    d. Bone marrow depression

50. Schizoaffective disorder is treated with antipsychotic medications and may require antidepressants. Which of the following medications is an antidepressant?

    a. Diazepam (Valium)

    b. Phenytoin (Dilantin)

    c. Chlorpromazine (Thorazine)

    d. Paroxetine (Paxil)

51. An anticholinergic drug is one that blocks the effects of:

    a. Epinephrine

    b. Norepinephrine

    c. Acetylcholine

    d. Serotonin

52. Succinimides, barbiturates, and benzodiazepines are used to treat:

    a. Anxiety

    b. Seizures

    c. Sleep disorders

    d. Mood disorders

53. Which type of drug is given to discourage tardive dyskinesia in patients being treated for psychosis?

    a. Cholinergics

    b. Anticholinergics

    c. Dopaminergics

    d. Selective serotonin reuptake inhibitors

CASE STUDY APPLICATIONS

54. Ms. S has been taking Thorazine for about a year. She has been having problems with orthostatic hypotension and akathisia and has needed to take Cogentin to avoid dystonic reactions. The physician has decided to change her to Clozaril. The patient asks the nurse about the advantages and disadvantages of the new drug. The nurse has chosen knowledge deficit as the nursing diagnosis for this patient.

    a. What interventions would be used for this diagnosis?

    b. How would the nurse evaluate the outcome of the interventions?

55. Ms. G has recently been diagnosed with schizophrenia. She has been placed on Haldol while hospitalized and has had hallucinations and delusions. What assessments would the nurse need to complete during the first 3 weeks that the patient is on this medication?

CHAPTER 12

DRUGS FOR DEGENERATIVE DISEASES AND MUSCLES

LEARNING OUTCOMES

To view the objectives, please refer to the textbook or MyNursingKit™ at www.mynursingkit.com.

TRUE/FALSE

For Questions 1–9, choose T for true or F for false.

T F 1. Dopamine is the major neurotransmitter within the hippocampus, an area of the brain responsible for learning and memory.

T F 2. Current medications for Alzheimer's disease result in only minor improvement of symptoms.

T F 3. An inability to remember or recall information is among the early symptoms of Alzheimer's disease.

T F 4. The anticholinergic agents produce more side effects than the dopaminergic drugs; thus, their primary use is for patients who cannot tolerate levodopa.

T F 5. Multiple sclerosis (MS) is an autoimmune disorder of the central nervous system (CNS) in which antibodies target and slowly destroy unmyelinated tissues in the brain and spinal cord.

T F 6. Interferon beta-1a (Avonex, Rebif) and interferon beta-1b (Betaseron) are the only clinically proven treatments for affecting the underlying course of multiple sclerosis and for decreasing overall relapse rate.

T F 7. The goal of drug therapy for spasticity is to improve the patient's mobility.

T F 8. Botulinum toxin acts as a poison if given in high doses.

T F 9. Convulsions, or muscle spasms, are common in patients with severe hypocalcemia.

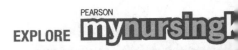

FILL IN THE BLANK

From the text, find the correct word(s) to complete the statement(s).

10. A patient with Parkinson's disease may experience difficulty urinating and performing sexually, which are signs of disturbances of the _____ nervous system.

11. Drug therapy for Parkinson's disease focuses on restoring dopamine function and blocking the effect of _____ within the same area of the brain.

12. _____ is a degenerative disorder characterized by progressive memory loss, confusion, and an inability to think or communicate effectively.

13. The most common causes of dementia are _____ and _____.

14. Patients with Alzheimer's disease experience a dramatic loss of their ability to perform tasks that require _____ as a neurotransmitter.

15. Parkinson's disease could have a _____ link, because many patients have a family history of the disorder.

16. Extensive treatment with certain _____ medications may induce Parkinson-like syndrome or _____ symptoms.

17. Side effects of drugs used to treat parkinsonism include _____ and _____. Signs of toxicity include _____ and _____.

18. When treating Alzheimer's disease, the goal of pharmacotherapy is to improve the function in three domains: _____, _____, and _____.

19. _____ can be used only in the early stages of Alzheimer's disease because they are effective only in the presence of _____ neurons.

20. Involuntary contractions of a muscle or group of muscles are called _____.

21. Pharmacotherapy used for muscle spasm usually includes _____, _____, and _____ drugs.

22. A muscle condition that results from damage to the CNS is _____.

23. A chronic neurologic disorder in which involuntary muscle contraction forces body parts into abnormal postures is _____.

24. Prolonged muscle spasms are referred to as _____.

MATCHING

For Questions 25–34, match the drug in Column I with its primary classification in Column II.

Column I	Column II
25. _____ Biperiden hydrochloride (Akineton)	a. Dopaminergic drug
26. _____ Levodopa (L-Dopa, Larodopa)	b. Cholinergic blocking drug
27. _____ Tacrine (Cognex)	c. Cholinergic drug (AchE inhibitor)
28. _____ Pergolide (Permax)	
29. _____ Benztropine (Cogentin)	
30. _____ Donepezil (Aricept)	
31. _____ Bromocriptine (Parlodel)	
32. _____ Tolcapone (Tasmar)	
33. _____ Procyclidine (Kemadrin)	
34. _____ Galantamine (Reminyl)	

For Questions 35–43, match the characteristic in Column I with its drug in Column II.

Column I	Column II
35. _____ Decreases the effect of dopaminergics	a. Levodopa
36. _____ Antioxidant possibly useful in Alzheimer's disease	b. Sinemet
37. _____ Approved in Europe for dementia but not yet in the United States; can react with anticoagulants	c. Selegiline
	d. Bromocriptine
38. _____ Antiviral that releases dopamine from its nerve terminals	e. Amantadine
	f. Tacrine
39. _____ Acetylcholinesterase inhibitor used for Alzheimer's disease associated with hepatotoxicity	g. Ginkgo biloba
	h. Donepezil
40. _____ Drug of choice for parkinsonism	i. Pyridoxine
41. _____ Inhibits enzymes that destroy levodopa or dopamine	
42. _____ Dopamine agent that activates dopamine receptors	
43. _____ Carbidopa that is added to levodopa to make more levodopa available to enter the CNS	

For Questions 44–51, match the drug in Column I with its classification in Column II.

Column I	Column II
44. _____ Cyclobenzaprine (Flexeril)	a. Centrally acting antispasmodic
45. _____ Dantrolene (Dantrium)	b. Skeletal muscle relaxer
46. _____ Quinine sulfate (Quinamm)	
47. _____ Diazepam (Valium)	
48. _____ Chlorzoxazone (Parafon Forte)	
49. _____ Botulinum toxin A (Botox)	
50. _____ Carisoprodol (Soma)	
51. _____ Methocarbamol (Robaxin)	

MULTIPLE CHOICE

52. Parkinson's disease is a degenerative disorder of the nervous system caused by the death of neurons that produce:

    a. Dopamine

    b. Norepinephrine

    c. Acetylcholine

    d. Serotonin

53. A patient is admitted with a new diagnosis of Parkinson's disease. If the patient is in the early stages, what would usually NOT be seen on assessment?

    a. Tremor

    b. Muscle rigidity and weakness

    c. Bradykinesia

    d. Dementia

54. What is the relationship between acetylcholine and dopamine in the area of the brain that affects balance, posture, and involuntary muscle movement?

    a. Both dopamine and acetylcholine stimulate this region.

    b. Both dopamine and acetylcholine inhibit this region.

    c. Dopamine stimulates and acetylcholine inhibits this region.

    d. Dopamine inhibits and acetylcholine stimulates this region.

55. What class of drugs may induce artificial parkinsonism by interfering with the same neural pathway and functions modified by a lack of dopamine?

    a. Phenothiazines

    b. Tricyclic antidepressants

    c. MAO inhibitors

    d. Benzodiazepines

56. Which drug has been prescribed more extensively than any other drug for patients with Parkinson's disease?

    a. Carbidopa (Lodosyn)

    b. Benztropine (Cogentin)

    c. Levodopa (Larodopa)

    d. Tacrine (Cognex)

57. A patient is started on levodopa for Parkinson's disease. What type of side effects would be expected?

    a. Sleep disorders such as insomnia

    b. Sedation

    c. Involuntary muscle movements

    d. Seizures

58. If a patient is unable to tolerate dopaminergic medications, which class of drugs would likely be prescribed?

    a. Cholinergic drugs

    b. Anticholinergic drugs

    c. Antipsychotic drugs

    d. Selective serotonin reuptake inhibitors (SSRIs)

59. What normally causes vascular dementia?

    a. Multiple strokes

    b. Multiple heart attacks

    c. Too little blood flow to the brain

    d. Lack of sufficient neurotransmitters in certain areas of the brain

60. Amyloid plaques and neurofibrillary tangles within the brain are diagnostic signs of which of the following?

    a. Parkinson's disease

    b. Tardive dyskinesia

    c. Vascular dementia

    d. Alzheimer's disease

61. Acetylcholine inhibitors enhance the action of what chemical in the brain?

    a. Dopamine

    b. Norepinephrine

    c. Acetylcholine

    d. Serotonin

62. Drugs that inhibit the enzyme acetylcholinesterase (AchE):

   a. Increase levels of dopamine

   b. Decrease levels of dopamine

   c. Increase levels of acetylcholine

   d. Decrease levels of acetylcholine

63. Causes of muscle spasms include all of the following EXCEPT:

   a. Overmedication with antipsychotic drugs

   b. Overdose of calcium

   c. Hypocalcemia

   d. Epilepsy

64. Nonpharmacologic measures that may be used to treat muscle spasms include all of the following EXCEPT:

   a. Use of the affected muscle

   b. Thermotherapy

   c. Hydrotherapy

   d. Ultrasound

65. Which of the following statements about cyclobenzaprine (Flexeril) is false?

   a. Its mechanism of action is similar to that of tricyclic antidepressants.

   b. It is effective in cerebral palsy.

   c. It is meant for short-term use.

   d. It is not recommended for use in children.

66. All of the following drugs are effective in the treatment of spasticity EXCEPT:

   a. Baclofen

   b. Diazepam

   c. Dantrolene

   d. Cyclobenzaprine

67. How does botulinum toxin (Botox, Myobloc) produce its effects?

   a. It blocks the release of norepinephrine from nerve tissue.

   b. It blocks the release of acetylcholine from cholinergic nerve terminals.

   c. It increases the release of acetylcholine from cholinergic nerve terminals.

   d. It increases the rate at which GABA is broken down in the body.

68. When teaching a patient receiving a centrally acting antispasmodic drug, which statement is INCORRECT?

   a. "You should avoid hazardous activities, such as driving, if the drug makes you drowsy."

   b. "You should avoid alcohol and antihistamines."

   c. "If you have severe side effects, stop taking the drug at once."

   d. "You should not take this drug if you have liver disease."

69. All of the following statements regarding dantrolene (Dantrium) are correct EXCEPT:

    a. Its use is contraindicated in patients with malignant hyperthermia.

    b. It is useful in spasms of head and neck muscles.

    c. It is useful in cases of spinal cord injury or CVA.

    d. It does not affect cardiac or smooth muscle.

70. Which of the following statements best describes the etiology of tetany?

    a. Blood calcium levels are too low, leading to cell membranes being extremely excitable.

    b. Blood calcium levels are too high, leading to cell membranes being extremely excitable.

    c. Blood potassium levels are too low, leading to cell membranes being extremely excitable.

    d. Blood calcium levels are too low, leading to cell membranes being extremely lethargic.

71. Which of the following drugs is produced by bacteria and is responsible for food poisoning in high quantities?

    a. Dantrolene

    b. Botulinum toxin

    c. Quinine sulfate

    d. Diazepam

72. Which of the following drug classes increases the risk for unfavorable reactions to antispasmodics?

    a. MAO inhibitors

    b. Pain medications

    c. Antibiotics

    d. Anticonvulsants

73. Patients who abruptly discontinue baclofen (Lioresal) may experience which of the following?

    a. Palpitations, chest pain, dyspnea

    b. Urinary retention

    c. Hallucinations, paranoia, and seizures

    d. Dry mouth and photosensitivity

74. A patient reports that, in addition to the drug therapy provided by his nurse, he is using cayenne (*Capsicum annum*) for his muscle spasms. Which precaution should this patient take?

    a. Wear sun block lotion and long sleeves.

    b. Never apply to broken skin.

    c. Do not use this substance if using any alcohol.

    d. If you notice any urinary hesitancy, discontinue use at once.

DO YOU REMEMBER?

75. Patients on herbal supplements must be warned about interactions with prescribed medications. What herbal preparation is sometimes taken to treat mental illness?

    a. Tryptophan

    b. St. John's wort

    c. Kava kava

    d. All of the above

76. An anticholinergic drug is one that blocks the effects of:

    a. Epinephrine

    b. Norepinephrine

    c. Acetylcholine

    d. Serotonin

77. Tacrine is highly metabolized by the liver. During the process of metabolism, what happens to the medication?

    a. It is absorbed into the bloodstream.

    b. It is excreted from the body.

    c. It is added to plasma proteins.

    d. It is made more or less active.

78. Antipsychotic medications have actions that decrease which of the following in the brain?

    a. Dopamine

    b. Acetylcholine

    c. Norepinephrine

    d. Acetylcholinesterase

CASE STUDY APPLICATIONS

79. Mr. H is a 30-year-old patient who has recently been diagnosed with early Parkinson's disease. He has been quite upset and depressed about the diagnosis and has lost interest in most of his usual activities and hobbies. His wife reports that his tremors and involuntary movements have worsened. He has been taking the following medications for 6 months: levodopa (2 g/day) and sertraline (Zoloft). He now has Cogentin added to his medications.

    a. What is the nursing diagnosis that best describes problems related to his condition and his new medication?

    b. What goal would relate to the diagnosis?

80. Mr. B has been brought to your facility by his wife. He was diagnosed last year with Alzheimer's disease. His confusion has become increasingly worse. He has been restless and agitated and has been experiencing hallucinations. This past year, he has been taking moderate doses of amitriptyline (Elavil) and alprazolam (Xanax). The patient is now placed on donepezil (Aricept) for a trial. During the first 4 weeks of the treatment with this AchE inhibitor, monitoring for adverse reactions and effectiveness is the responsibility of the nurse.

    a. What would be the priority nursing diagnosis for this situation?

    b. What interventions would be included?

81. Ms. H has been experiencing lower back pain for 2 months due to muscle spasms. So far, no other disorders have been identified that could explain this pain. Her doctor has prescribed cyclobenzaprine (Flexeril).

    a. Describe other nondrug therapy that might help in this case.

    b. When teaching Ms. H about adverse reactions to cyclobenzaprine, what information should be included?

    c. How will the nurse determine whether this drug is effective?

    d. Prior to discharge, your goal is to have the patient state ways to prevent recurrence of her symptoms. What preventive teaching should be done for this patient?

82. Your patient, Ms. B, has a career as a model and fashion designer. She expresses concern over the "crow's feet and frown lines" she is beginning to develop. She asks for information on the new Botox injections she has heard about. She expresses concern over the fact that she has heard they use a "poison" to remove facial wrinkles but says, "It would be great to look 16 again!" Your nursing diagnosis is knowledge deficit related to use of cosmetic procedures, and teaching is a planned intervention.

    a. What misinformation do you need to correct when talking with this patient?

    b. What side effects does Ms. B need to be aware of before having Botox injections?

83. Mr. P is a 21-year-old patient with cerebral palsy who is cared for at home by his parents. His mother expresses concern over his spasticity and wants "better drugs" to control it. He is currently using Lioresal.

    a. What assessments should be done on Mr. P?

    b. What nondrug therapy might be useful for Mr. P?

    c. What patient/family teaching should be done regarding Mr. P's use of antispasmodic drugs at home?

    d. What patient/family teaching should be done regarding nondrug and safety interventions for Mr. P?

CHAPTER 13

DRUGS FOR SEIZURES

LEARNING OUTCOMES

To view the objectives, please refer to the textbook or
MyNursingKit™ at www.mynursingkit.com.

TRUE/FALSE

For Questions 1–8, choose T for true or F for false.

T   F   1. Clients with epilepsy may appear normal and
asymptomatic.

T   F   2. The goal of antiseizure medication is to completely
suppress neuronal activity in the brain.

T   F   3. Status epilepticus is a medical emergency brought on by repeated seizures and convulsions.

T   F   4. Abnormal mineral fluxes and blood glucose or protein levels may explain the occurrence of most
seizures during pregnancy or childbirth.

T   F   5. Drugs that stimulate an influx of chloride ion across neuronal cell membranes are associated with the
neurotransmitter gamma-aminobutyric acid (GABA).

T   F   6. Some antiseizure medications may influence the rate of drug metabolism, decreasing the effectiveness of
other drug therapies.

T   F   7. Phenytoin (Dilantin) and carbamazepine (Tegretol) are useful for the treatment of partial seizures.

T   F   8. In severe cases of alcohol withdrawal, patients may experience seizures; however, antiseizure medication
is generally not given due to interactions with alcohol in the patient's bloodstream.

EXPLORE PEARSON 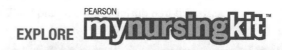 mynursingkit™

FILL IN THE BLANK

From the text, find the correct word(s) to complete the statement(s).

9. Seizures can result from _____ situations or occur on a(n) _____ basis, as with epilepsy.

10. Five possible causes of seizures are _____, _____, _____, _____, and _____.

11. Because antiseizure drugs are mostly pregnancy category D, patients should use _____ or other contraceptive measures.

12. Antiseizure drugs may cause _____ deficiency, which can cause neural tube defects in a fetus.

13. Patients who have seizures may have a lower tolerance to environmental triggers, such as _____ deprivation and exposure to _____ or _____ lights.

14. _____ seizures occur in 0.5% of _____ month-old to _____-year-old children during an illness and last 1 to 2 minutes. Prevention is best carried out by controlling _____.

15. Of the major antiseizure medications, _____ is a drug of choice for a broader range of seizure types.

16. _____ seizures occur only on one side of the brain and continue for a short distance before they stop; _____ seizures may travel throughout the brain.

17. Of the most popular antiseizure medications, the drug of choice for absence seizures is _____.

18. Two popular medications used to treat status epilepticus are _____ and _____.

19. _____ is an emergency type of generalized tonic-clonic seizure that is prolonged and usually affects _____, causing hypoxia.

20. If not treated, status epilepticus can cause _____ damage or death.

21. Treatment of status epilepticus includes maintenance of the _____ and IV antiseizure medications.

22. Abrupt discontinuation of antiseizure medications could cause _____.

23. The goal of antiseizure medications is to prevent _____ or repeated firing and, therefore, to _____ neuronal activity.

24. Once seizures are controlled, drug therapy continues for some time. After _____ years, the medications may be withdrawn slowly, one at a time, over several _____.

MATCHING

For Questions 25–31, match the sign and symptom in Column I with its type of seizure in Column II.

<table>
<tr><td>**Column I**</td><td>**Column II**</td></tr>
</table>

25. _____ In adults, this seizure may be preceded by an aura. Muscles then become tense, and a rhythmic jerking motion develops.

26. _____ This seizure is marked by major muscle groups contracting quickly, making a jerking motion. Patients appear unsteady and clumsy and may fall from a sitting position or drop whatever they are holding.

27. _____ This seizure usually starts with a blank stare. Patients may become disoriented and not pay attention to verbal commands or act as if they have a psychiatric illness. After the seizure, patients do not remember what happened.

28. _____ Patients may feel for a brief moment that their precise location is vague and out of sorts. Often, patients hear and see things that are not there or smell or taste things and have an upset stomach. Parts of the body, such as the arms, legs, or face, may start twitching. Symptoms are often not dramatic and may occur without loss of consciousness.

29. _____ This type of seizure occurs most often in children. Patients develop a blank stare without having twitching facial or body movements. This seizure lasts for only a few seconds. Patients then quickly recover and engage in normal activities.

30. _____ This is a medical emergency brought on by repeated seizures and convulsions. Steps must be taken to ensure that the airway remains open.

31. _____ Patients often stumble or fall for no apparent reason. Episodes are very short, lasting only seconds. After the seizure, patients return to normal activities without difficulty.

a. Simple partial seizure

b. Complex partial seizure (psychomotor or temporal lobe seizure)

c. Absence seizure (petit mal seizure)

d. Atonic seizure (drop attack)

e. Myoclonic seizure

f. Generalized tonic-clonic seizure (grand mal seizure)

g. Status epilepticus

For Questions 32–37, match the drug in Column I with its pharmacologic category in Column II.

Column I

32. _____ Phenobarbital (Luminal)

33. _____ Clonazepam (Klonopin)

34. _____ Phenytoin (Dilantin)

35. _____ Gabapentin (Neurontin)

36. _____ Carbamazepine (Tegretol)

37. _____ Ethosuximide (Zarontin)

Column II

a. Drugs acting through a GABA receptor

b. Drugs delaying an influx of sodium across neuronal membranes

c. Drugs delaying an influx of calcium across neuronal membranes

MULTIPLE CHOICE

38. What common concern occurs with phenobarbital (Luminal)?

    a. Irregular heartbeat

    b. Blood cell reactions

    c. Hypotension

    d. Vitamin D and folate deficiency

39. What is the main advantage of using carbamazepine (Tegretol) for partial seizures?

    a. Category C status

    b. Dual use for the treatment of trigeminal neuralgia

    c. Ability to cause less drowsiness

    d. Dual use for the treatment of bipolar disorder

40. Which one of the following is the newest hydantoin-like drug?

    a. Phenytoin (Dilantin)

    b. Zonisamide (Zonegran)

    c. Carbamazepine (Tegretol)

    d. Valproic acid (Depakene)

41. Which of the following medications is used to treat Lennox-Gastaut syndrome?

    a. Fosphenytoin (Cerebyx)

    b. Felbamate (Felbatol)

    c. Lamotrigine (Lamictal)

    d. Methsuximide (Celontin)

42. Which antiseizure medication might produce psychotic behavior symptoms?

    a. Ethosuximide (Zarontin)

    b. Amobarbital (Amytal)

    c. Lorazepam (Ativan)

    d. Gabapentin (Neurontin)

43. Which is the most potent benzodiazepine used for the treatment of convulsions?

    a. Clonazepam (Klonopin)

    b. Clorazepate (Tranxene)

    c. Diazepam (Valium)

    d. Lorazepam (Ativan)

44. Which of the following medications is converted to phenytoin in the body?

    a. Fosphenytoin (Cerebyx)

    b. Felbamate (Felbatol)

    c. Divalproex (Depakote)

    d. Lamotrigine (Lamictal)

45. What is the major concern in making antiseizure therapy successful?

    a. Avoiding kidney and liver toxicity

    b. Making sure that the patient complies with medication

    c. Maintaining proper drug levels in the bloodstream

    d. All of the above

46. Why should women of childbearing age be counseled regarding antiseizure medications?

    a. They are teratogenic.

    b. They interfere with oral contraceptives.

    c. They produce folic acid deficiency.

    d. All of the above are correct.

47. Patients taking barbiturates for seizures must be monitored for respiratory depression in the presence of:

    a. Oral administration

    b. Nonopiate analgesics

    c. Chronic respiratory dysfunction

    d. All of the above

48. A patient is admitted with an overdose of Valium. Which of the following drugs would the nurse need to have on hand?

    a. Diphenhydramine (Benadryl)

    b. Flumazenil (Romazicon)

    c. Epinephrine

    d. Atropine

49. The nurse should teach the patient taking benzodiazepines that the drug can do which of the following?

    a. Cause sedation when first started

    b. Be safely stopped abruptly

    c. Increase the amount of digoxin needed

    d. Be potentiated by smoking, nicotine patches, or chewing tobacco

50. A patient taking phenytoin (Dilantin) chronically for seizures should be encouraged to maintain good oral hygiene and visit the dentist every 6 months. Phenytoin does which of the following in patients?

    a. Causes cavities

    b. Causes gingival hyperplasia

    c. Causes mouth cancers

    d. Builds up tartar on the teeth

DO YOU REMEMBER?

51. Although phenobarbital is an antiseizure medicine, it is also classified a:

    a. Benzodiazepine

    b. Category I drug

    c. Sympathomimetic

    d. Sedative-hypnotic

52. A patient's craving to continue drug use despite its negative effects is:

    a. Tolerance

    b. Physical dependence

    c. Psychological dependence

    d. Resistance

53. When are seizures in a patient who is undergoing alcohol withdrawal most likely to occur?

    a. Immediately after the patient has stopped drinking

    b. 1 to 3 days after the patient has stopped drinking

    c. 5 to 7 days after the patient has stopped drinking

    d. During an episode of delirium tremens (DTs)

54. Which of the following drugs is not used to treat convulsions?

    a. Buspirone (BuSpar)

    b. Phenobarbital (Luminal)

    c. Gabapentin (Neurontin)

    d. Carbamazepine (Tegretol)

55. What is the most important reason benzodiazepines are not used for chronic seizure control?

    a. Patients tend to develop tolerance to the drug.

    b. Patients are likely to develop psychological addiction.

    c. Respiratory depression occurs with chronic use.

    d. No antidote exists.

CASE STUDY APPLICATIONS

56. A nurse is preparing for a patient who is coming to the emergency department (ED) with status epilepticus. The physician has ordered Dilantin by IV drip as soon as the patient arrives.

    a. What evidence (assessment data) would support a nursing diagnosis of "Risk for injury"?

    b. What interventions would provide safety for the patient during Dilantin administration?

57. A male patient has been placed on Dilantin for newly diagnosed epilepsy. He has generalized tonic-clonic seizures. He has asked how long it will take to manage his seizures and what side effects can occur. He also wants to know what foods or drugs to avoid while on this medication.

    a. Which nursing diagnosis would be top priority for this patient?

    b. What interventions would be helpful for this diagnosis?

CHAPTER 14

DRUGS FOR PAIN CONTROL

LEARNING OUTCOMES

To view the objectives, please refer to the textbook or
MyNursingKit™ at www.mynursingkit.com.

TRUE/FALSE

For Questions 1–9, choose T for true or F for false.

T F 1. The perception of pain and the psychological reaction to
pain are nearly the same for every patient.

T F 2. The sensation of pain is almost entirely emotional in
nature and has very little physiologic basis.

T F 3. A fibers signal sharp, well-defined pain, whereas C fibers conduct dull, poorly localized pain.

T F 4. All analgesics are also able to reduce fever.

T F 5. Acetaminophen (Tylenol) should not be used for children experiencing fever, chickenpox, or influenza-
like symptoms.

T F 6. Because aspirin increases bleeding time, it should not be given with anticoagulants.

T F 7. In medical environments, the term *narcotic* should be used to refer to abused illegal drugs, such as
hallucinogens, heroin, amphetamines, and marijuana.

T F 8. Fever is a normal sign of the body's defense system attempting to remove foreign organisms.

T F 9. Selection of the correct analgesic is dependent on the nature and character of the pain.

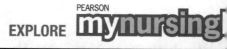

FILL IN THE BLANK

From the text, find the correct word(s) to complete the statement(s).

10. The two main classes of pain medications are the _____ and the _____.

11. All nonsteroidal anti-inflammatory drugs (NSAIDs) have _____ and _____ activity as well as analgesic properties.

12. The narcotic analgesics are obtained from _____.

13. A headache characterized by a tightening of the muscles of the head and neck area due to stress is called a _____ headache.

14. A sensory cue that precedes a migraine is called a(n) _____.

15. NSAIDs act by inhibiting pain mediators at the _____ level.

16. The sensation of pain is increased by _____, _____, and _____.

17. The successful choice of pain therapy is dependent on the _____ and _____ of the pain.

18. The goals of pharmacotherapy for migraine are to _____ the migraine in progress and to _____ migraines from occurring.

19. Two major drug classes used for migraine headaches are _____ and _____. Both of these are _____ agonists.

20. Triptans are 5-HT-selective and are thought to act by constricting _____. They are available to be administered _____, _____, or _____.

MATCHING

For Questions 21–32, match the drug in Column I with its primary indication/class in Column II.

Column I	Column II
21. _____ Naloxone (Narcan)	a. NSAID
22. _____ Meperidine (Demerol)	b. Opioid; moderate effectiveness
23. _____ Celecoxib (Celebrex)	c. Opioid; high effectiveness
24. _____ Oxycodone (OxyContin)	d. Opioid blocker
25. _____ Zolmitriptan (Zomig)	e. Antimigraine agent
26. _____ Nalmefene (Revex)	
27. _____ Ibuprofen (Advil, Motrin)	
28. _____ Ergotamine tartrate (Ergostat)	
29. _____ Oxymorphone (Numorphan)	
30. _____ Fenoprofen (Nalfon)	
31. _____ Propranolol (Inderal)	
32. _____ Amitriptyline (Elavil)	

For Questions 33–38, match the description in Column I with its related term in Column II.

<table>
<tr><td>Column I</td><td>Column II</td></tr>
</table>

Column I	Column II
33. _____ Natural or synthetic chemicals providing pain relief	a. Nociceptor pain
	b. Neuropathic pain
34. _____ Dull, throbbing, or aching pain	c. Somatic pain
35. _____ Caused by injury to tissues	d. Visceral pain
36. _____ Sharp, localized pain	e. Opiates
37. _____ Caused by injury to nerves	f. Opioids
38. _____ Natural chemicals that relieve pain	

MULTIPLE CHOICE

39. Painful disorders having a strong inflammatory component, such as arthritis, are treated most effectively with:

    a. NSAIDs

    b. Acetaminophen (Tylenol)

    c. Opioids

    d. Herbal supplements

40. When asked why NSAIDs are better than acetaminophen for arthritis, the health care provider responds, "Compared with aspirin, acetaminophen has:_____."

    a. Less analgesic activity

    b. No antipyretic activity

    c. No anti-inflammatory activity

    d. The same effect on blood coagulation

41. Which of the following would be used to treat mild to moderate pain due to inflammation?

    a. Oxycodone (OxyContin)

    b. Meperidine (Demerol)

    c. Ibuprofen (Advil)

    d. Acetaminophen (Tylenol)

42. Why are selective COX-2 inhibitors often prescribed over aspirin?

    a. They are more effective at relieving severe pain.

    b. They are more effective at relieving dull, throbbing pain.

    c. They are less expensive.

    d. They cause fewer side effects.

43. ASA is an abbreviation that refers to which of the following?

    a. Any NSAID

    b. Aspirin

    c. Opioid analgesics

    d. COX-2 inhibitors

44. A health care provider sees an order for aspirin 325 mg once daily. The health care provider knows that this medication is given at this dose level for what reason?

    a. To prolong clotting times

    b. To fight infections

    c. To relieve pain

    d. To decrease inflammation

45. When a health care provider is asked to explain why Tylenol is used more often than aspirin, the response is that aspirin can cause:

    a. Dependence

    b. Increased platelet adhesiveness

    c. Gastrointestinal (GI) bleeding

    d. Central nervous system (CNS) depression

46. A mother asks why aspirin should not be given to children and teens. The appropriate reaction by the health care provider is based on the actions of aspirin, which can cause:

    a. Anticoagulant activity

    b. Reduced incidence of strokes

    c. Reduced risk of colorectal cancer

    d. Increased risk of Reye's syndrome

47. Which of the following drugs is commonly given to heroin addicts during treatment of their drug dependence?

    a. Methadone (Dolophine)

    b. Oxycodone

    c. Morphine

    d. Meperidine (Demerol)

48. Why are opioids often used for pain relief following tooth extractions?

    a. They help the client sleep.

    b. They do not prolong bleeding time.

    c. They can be taken once a day.

    d. They are more effective than other analgesics.

49. A health care provider knows that the therapeutic effects of opiates do NOT include:

    a. Treatment of respiratory depression

    b. Treatment of diarrhea

    c. Relief of severe pain

    d. Suppression of cough reflex

50. A client goes to the emergency department (ED) with an overdose of morphine. What would the priority nursing assessment include?

    a. Dilated pupils

    b. Depressed respiration

    c. Hypertension

    d. Diarrhea

51. What would the health care provider need to have on hand to counteract the effects of an overdose of opiates?

    a. Dextroamphetamine (Dexedrine)

    b. Phenytoin (Dilantin)

    c. Naloxone (Narcan)

    d. Tramadol (Ultram)

52. A patient goes to the ED with complaints of symptoms resembling an aura. The health care provider knows that the patient may have an aura prior to the onset of a migraine. What does the aura indicate about the patient?

    a. The patient has taken an overdose of aspirin.

    b. The patient has taken an overdose of opioids.

    c. The patient may soon be experiencing a seizure.

    d. The patient has a high fever.

53. What is the mechanism of action of sumatriptan (Imitrex) and other triptans?

    a. They affect mu receptors.

    b. They cause vasoconstriction of cranial arteries.

    c. They block prostaglandin synthesis.

    d. They block COX-2.

DO YOU REMEMBER?

54. Besides an antimigraine agent, what is another use for amitriptyline?

    a. Anticonvulsant

    b. Sedative-hypnotic

    c. Antipsychotic

    d. Antidepressant

55. Ergotamine is a category X drug, which means that it:

    a. Has a high risk of physical and psychological dependence

    b. Should never be taken during pregnancy

    c. Has no therapeutic use

    d. Is very toxic to the patient

56. Phenobarbital (Luminal) is a sedative-hypnotic that is also prescribed for:

    a. Migraines

    b. Marijuana addiction

    c. Seizures

    d. Clinical depression

57. Where would an intrathecal injection of morphine be administered?

    a. Spinal subarachnoid space

    b. Brain

    c. Joint

    d. Abdominal cavity

58. What is the first step in pharmacokinetics?

    a. Metabolism

    b. Absorption

    c. Ingestion

    d. Excretion

CASE STUDY APPLICATIONS

59. Mr. T arrives in your office, complaining of severe pain in his joints. You, as his nurse, are asked to assess his complaints and recommend a course of treatment. He is 75 years old and, other than anxiety and insomnia, appears to be in good health. Mr. T is interested in nonpharmacologic control of his pain. He admits to being reluctant to take the oxycodone that the physician ordered, because he does not want to "become a crazy addict." Past records indicate a nursing diagnosis of "Knowledge deficit."

    a. What interventions would be appropriate for this situation?

    b. What outcomes would be evaluated for this patient?

60. Ms. M has been experiencing migraine headaches for 2 years. She is now seeking medical assistance because they have become more frequent and painful. She states that it takes six aspirin to relieve the pain once the migraine has started. She has a history of chronic heart failure and hypertension. She has heard that drugs used for migraines are addictive and is interested in a nonpharmacologic solution. The following medications are being taken:

    Oxycodone terephthalate (Percodan) (as needed)
    Verapamil (Calan)
    Digoxin (Lanoxin)

    a. The nurse chooses altered comfort: pain as the diagnosis. What interventions can be used for this nursing diagnosis?

    b. What patient goals would be included in the care for this patient?

CHAPTER 15

DRUGS FOR ANESTHESIA

LEARNING OUTCOMES

To view the objectives, please refer to the textbook or MyNursingKit™ at www.mynursingkit.com.

TRUE/FALSE

For Questions 1–6, choose T for true or F for false.

T F 1. Drugs used to produce general anesthesia are the same as those for local anesthesia, except higher doses are administered.

T F 2. General anesthesia usually results in a loss of consciousness.

T F 3. Because the blocking of ion channels during local anesthesia is a nonselective process, only sensory impulses are affected, leaving motor impulses unaffected.

T F 4. Cocaine was the first local anesthetic discovered, and it is still widely used for eye surgery.

T F 5. Allergy to local anesthetic medications is common.

T F 6. Halothane (Fluothane) is often used with other anesthetic agents, including muscle relaxants and analgesics, because it has low potency and is unable to induce surgical anesthesia.

FILL IN THE BLANK

From the text, find the correct word(s) to complete the statement(s).

7. Because local anesthesia is not always applied to small areas of the body, some local anesthetic treatments are more accurately called _____ anesthesia.

8. The direct injection of a local anesthetic into tissue immediate to a surgical site is called _____ anesthesia.

 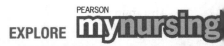

9. The goal of general anesthesia is to provide a rapid and complete loss of _____.

10. The two major ways to induce general anesthesia are by using _____ agents and _____ agents.

11. Opioids are sometimes given as preoperative medications to counteract _____.

12. Local anesthesia is loss of _____ to a small area without loss of _____.

13. In applying local anesthesia, the method employed depends on _____ and _____.

14. In the area where the local anesthetic is applied, _____ and _____ will temporarily diminish.

15. Drug classes used as adjuncts to anesthesia include _____, _____, _____, and _____.

16. The advantage of _____ anesthesia is that the dose of anesthetic can be _____, thus making the procedure safer for the patient.

MATCHING

For Questions 17–29, match the drug in Column I with its classification in Column II.

Column I	**Column II**
17. _____ Droperidol (Inapsine)	a. Ester-type local anesthetic
18. _____ Benzocaine (Anbesol)	b. Amide-type local anesthetic
19. _____ Bupivacaine (Marcaine)	c. Inhaled anesthetic
20. _____ Enflurane (Ethrane)	d. Intravenous anesthetic
21. _____ Diazepam (Valium)	e. Adjunct to anesthesia
22. _____ Lidocaine (Xylocaine)	
23. _____ Prilocaine (Citanest)	
24. _____ Fentanyl (Duragesic, Actiq, others) – two answers are correct	
25. _____ Promethazine (Phenergan, others)	
26. _____ Ketamine (Ketalar)	
27. _____ Isoflurane (Forane)	
28. _____ Pentobarbital (Nembutal)	
29. _____ Thiopental (Pentothal)	

For Questions 30–38, match the characteristic in Column I with its drug or class in Column II.

<table>
<tr><td colspan="2">**Column I**</td><td>**Column II**</td></tr>
<tr><td>30. _____</td><td>Prolongs duration of local anesthetic agents</td><td>a. Epinephrine</td></tr>
<tr><td>31. _____</td><td>Most commonly used topical anesthetic</td><td>b. Epidural</td></tr>
<tr><td>32. _____</td><td>May be prescribed for cardiac dysrhythmias</td><td>c. Amides</td></tr>
<tr><td>33. _____</td><td>Type of anesthesia most commonly used in obstetrics (OB) during labor and delivery</td><td>d. Benzocaine
e. Lidocaine
f. Isoflurane (Forane)</td></tr>
<tr><td>34. _____</td><td>Most commonly used injectable local anesthetic</td><td>g. Succinylcholine</td></tr>
<tr><td>35. _____</td><td>Most commonly used local anesthetic</td><td>h. Nitrous oxide</td></tr>
<tr><td>36. _____</td><td>Most abused anesthetic agent</td><td></td></tr>
<tr><td>37. _____</td><td>Major depolarizing neuromuscular blocker</td><td></td></tr>
<tr><td>38. _____</td><td>Most widely used inhalation anesthesia</td><td></td></tr>
</table>

MULTIPLE CHOICE

39. Epinephrine is often added to a local anesthetic. The nurse must monitor for which factor when caring for the patient who is due to receive epinephrine in his anesthetic?

   a. Side effects of increased heart rate and blood pressure (BP)

   b. History of cardiac conditions

   c. Vital signs

   d. All of the above

40. Which of the following is NOT a major route for applying local anesthetics?

   a. Epidural

   b. Spinal

   c. Nerve block

   d. Inhalation

41. In administering general anesthetics using balanced anesthesia, the nurse would expect which medication to be administered first?

   a. IV anesthesia

   b. Inhalation anesthesia

   c. Analgesics

   d. Neuromuscular blocking agents

42. Nitrous oxide can be administered safely in patients with:

    a. Myasthenia gravis

    b. Increased anxiety related to pain or procedures

    c. Increased intracranial pressure

    d. Cardiac disease

43. An alkaline substance, such as sodium hydroxide, is sometimes added to a vial of anesthetic solution for what reason?

    a. To provide the environment needed for absorption

    b. To prolong the duration of anesthetic action

    c. To increase the effectiveness of the anesthetic in regions that have extensive local infection or abscesses

    d. To decrease the potential for anaphylaxis

44. Which of the following is a potential early adverse effect of local anesthetics?

    a. Hypertension

    b. Myocardial infarction

    c. Flushing

    d. Restlessness or anxiety

45. Which stage of general anesthesia is called surgical anesthesia because it is the stage in which most surgery occurs?

    a. Stage 1

    b. Stage 2

    c. Stage 3

    d. Stage 4

46. The *primary* reason nitrous oxide is used in dentistry is that it provides:

    a. Potent analgesia

    b. Sedation/relaxation

    c. Anti-inflammatory effects

    d. Anti-infective effects

47. Inhaled general anesthetics produce their effect by preventing the flow of which of the following into neurons of the central nervous system (CNS)?

    a. Carbohydrates

    b. Lipids

    c. Sodium

    d. Calcium

48. Which of the following is a potential early adverse effect of nitrous oxide?

    a. Restlessness or anxiety

    b. Dysrhythmia

    c. Hypertension

    d. Mania

49. What is the major depolarizing neuromuscular blocker used during surgery?

    a. Succinylcholine (Anectine)

    b. Acetylcholine

    c. Promethazine (Phenergan)

    d. Bethanechol (Urecholine)

50. Which of the following is a parasympathomimetic sometimes administered to stimulate the smooth muscle of the bowel and the urinary tract following surgery?

    a. Succinylcholine (Anectine)

    b. Acetylcholine

    c. Promethazine (Phenergan)

    d. Bethanechol (Urecholine)

51. Hepatitis can be prevented by using Halothane:

    a. In those presently not pregnant

    b. At least 21 days apart

    c. With caution in those having diminished hepatic function

    d. In those having high blood pressure or irregular heartbeats

DO YOU REMEMBER?

52. In addition to its use as an injected anesthetic, what is lorazepam (Ativan) also used to treat?

    a. Depression

    b. Anxiety

    c. Loss of appetite

    d. Bipolar disorder

53. Where are sublingual medications administered?

    a. Into a body cavity

    b. Into the subarachnoid spinal space

    c. Into a vein or an artery

    d. Under the tongue

54. Which of the following is a hallucinogen?

    a. Psilocybin

    b. Cocaine

    c. Heroin

    d. Marijuana

55. Before administering an opioid, which of the following should be checked?

    a. Blood pressure

    b. Respiration rate

    c. Body temperature

    d. Pulse rate

56. Adrenergic blockers produce a response similar to that of:

    a. Sympathetic stimulation

    b. Parasympathetic stimulation

    c. Dopaminergic inhibition

    d. Serotonin inhibition

CASE STUDY APPLICATIONS

57. Ms. K is to undergo a procedure that requires general anesthesia. She asks the nurse what to expect from the medications and before and after the procedure.

    a. Identify the nursing diagnosis.

    b. Describe interventions that would be appropriate for this patient.

58. Mrs. B is to have a minor procedure on her foot, during which local anesthesia is to be used. She is anxious and asks how this procedure is done. She asks what type of effect the anesthesia will have and how long the anesthesia will last. Mrs. B has rapid speech and talks in a pressured speech pattern. She is tremulous and seems to be restless, scanning the room frequently.

    a. Identify the nursing diagnosis.

    b. What assessment data would cause the nurse to have picked the diagnosis?

    c. Describe interventions that would be appropriate for this patient.

    d. Identify the goal(s) for this patient.

    e. How would each goal be evaluated by the nurse?

CHAPTER 16

DRUGS FOR LIPID DISORDERS

LEARNING OUTCOMES

To view the objectives, please refer to the textbook or MyNursingKit™ at www.mynursingkit.com.

TRUE/FALSE

For Questions 1–10, choose T for true or F for false.

T F 1. Cholesterol is the most common type of lipid, accounting for about 90% of all lipids in the body.

T F 2. The steroids are a diverse group of lipids, having a common chemical group called the cholesterol nucleus or ring.

T F 3. Dietary cholesterol can only be obtained from animal food products.

T F 4. Very low-density lipoprotein (VLDL) is converted to low-density lipoprotein (LDL) as it travels through the bloodstream.

T F 5. When taking drugs for hyperlipidemia, it is desirable to maintain the level of low-density lipoproteins to 130 mg/dl or higher.

T F 6. In order to significantly reduce blood cholesterol levels, the patient must also limit the dietary intake of unsaturated fat.

T F 7. Ingestion of omega-3 fatty acids has been found to increase plaque formation and the potential for heart disease.

T F 8. The statins have been shown to slow the progression of coronary artery disease and to reduce mortality from cardiovascular disease.

T F 9. Many of the statins should be administered at breakfast, because cholesterol biosynthesis in the body is higher in the morning.

T F 10. The bile acid-binding drugs tend to cause more frequent adverse effects than the statins.

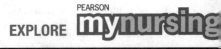

EXPLORE **mynursing**
PEARSON

www.mynursingkit.com

MyNursingKit is your one stop for online chapter review materials and resources. Prepare for success with additional NCLEX®-style practice questions, interactive assignments and activities, web links, animations and videos, and more! Register your access code from the front of your book at www.mynursingkit.com.

FILL IN THE BLANK

From the text, find the correct word(s) to complete the statement(s).

11. The general term that means high levels of lipids in the blood is _____.

12. Cholesterol contributes to the fatty _____ that narrows arteries.

13. The three basic types of lipids are _____, _____, and _____.

14. Lipoproteins consist of various amounts of _____, _____, and _____, along with a protein carrier.

15. The _____ class of antihyperlipidemics interferes with a critical enzyme in the synthesis of cholesterol.

16. The fibric acid agents have been largely replaced by the _____.

17. In the figure below, identify the drugs/drug classes:

    A. _____

    B. _____

    C. _____

    D. _____

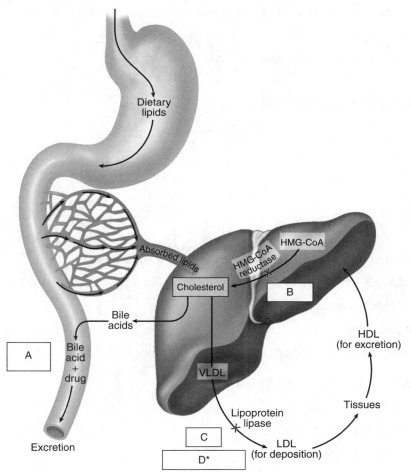

*Mechanism not completely understood

MATCHING

For Questions 18–22, match the drug in Column I with its primary class in Column II.

	Column I		**Column II**
18.	_____ Cholestyramine (Questran)	a.	HMG-CoA reductase inhibitor
19.	_____ Pravastatin (Pravachol)	b.	Bile acid-binding agent
20.	_____ Nicotinic acid	c.	Fibric acid agent
21.	_____ Gemfibrozil (Lopid)	d.	None of the above
22.	_____ Fluvastatin (Lescol)		

MULTIPLE CHOICE

23. Antihyperlipidemic agents are prescribed to reduce the likelihood of:

    a. Dysrhythmias

    b. Colon cancer

    c. Coronary artery disease

    d. Obesity

24. LDL transports cholesterol from the liver to the tissues and organs, where it is used to:

    a. Provide energy for cells

    b. Build plasma membranes or synthesize steroids

    c. Make bile

    d. Make high-density lipoprotein (HDL)

25. LDL is often called _____ cholesterol.

    a. Good

    b. Bad

    c. High

    d. Low

26. The cholesterol component of HDL is transported to the liver, where it is:

    a. Used to make LDL

    b. Used to build plasma membranes

    c. Used as an energy source

    d. Broken down to become part of bile

27. The goal in maintaining normal blood cholesterol levels is to:

    a. Minimize both HDL and LDL

    b. Maximize both HDL and LDL

    c. Maximize HDL and minimize LDL

    d. Maximize LDL and minimize HDL

28. Which of the following is NOT a lifestyle change that should be considered by patients with high blood lipid levels?

    a. Maintain weight at an optimum level.

    b. Implement a medically supervised exercise plan.

    c. Reduce sources of stress.

    d. Limit soluble fiber in the diet to 2 or fewer grams per day.

29. Which drugs are considered agents of first choice for reducing blood lipid levels?

    a. HMG-CoA reductase inhibitors

    b. Fibric acid agents

    c. Niacin

    d. Bile acid resins

30. Statins can produce a _____ reduction in LDL cholesterol levels.

    a. 5–10%

    b. 20–40%

    c. 50–60%

    d. 70–80%

31. HMG-CoA reductase serves as the primary regulatory enzyme for the biosynthesis of:

    a. Cholesterol

    b. Steroid hormones

    c. Triglycerides

    d. HDL

32. The statins act by:

    a. Binding bile acids

    b. Reducing bile synthesis in the liver

    c. Inhibiting HMG-CoA reductase

    d. Decreasing the absorption of dietary cholesterol

33. Maximum effects from atorvastatin (Lipitor) take _____ to achieve.

    a. 4 to 8 hours

    b. 2 weeks

    c. 4 to 8 weeks

    d. 3 to 4 months

34. Which of the following should be monitored carefully during the first few months of therapy with the statins?

    a. Blood pressure

    b. Sleep patterns

    c. Cardiac function

    d. Liver function

35. Bile acid resins produce their therapeutic effects by:

    a. Inhibiting HMG-CoA reductase

    b. Increasing excretion of cholesterol in the feces

    c. Decreasing production of HDL

    d. Decreasing absorption of dietary lipids

36. All of the following are true regarding cholestyramine (Questran) EXCEPT:

    a. It is not absorbed or metabolized once it enters the intestine.

    b. It acts by inhibiting cholesterol biosynthesis.

    c. Its most frequent adverse effects are constipation, bloating, gas, and nausea.

    d. It should not be taken at the same time as other medications.

37. Which of the following is a B-complex vitamin?

    a. Nicotinic acid

    b. Gemfibrozil (Lopid)

    c. Lovastatin (Mevacor)

    d. Colestipol (Colestid)

38. Which of the following best describes the use of nicotinic acid in treating hyperlipidemias?

    a. It should not be used in patients with hypercholesterolemia.

    b. It should not be used in patients with a history of heart failure.

    c. It should not be used with other antihyperlipidemics, because their effects may cancel out each other.

    d. It is most often used in lower doses in combination with a statin.

39. Which of the following best describes the use of the fibric acid agents in treating hyperlipidemias?

    a. They should always be given at least 2 hours before or after other medications.

    b. They should not be used in patients with a history of liver failure.

    c. They should not be used with other antihyperlipidemics, because their effects may cancel out each other.

    d. They are most often used in lower doses in combination with a statin.

40. Which of the following should be taken separately from other medications, because it may interfere with drug absorption?

    a. Nicotinic acid

    b. Gemfibrozil (Lopid)

    c. Cholestyramine (Questran)

    d. Fluvastatin (Lescol)

DO YOU REMEMBER?

41. Which of the following best describes acetaminophen (Tylenol)?

    a. Opioid

    b. Analgesic

    c. Anti-inflammatory

    d. NSAID

42. ALL of the following are therapeutic effects of aspirin EXCEPT:

    a. Increased prothrombin time

    b. Prevention of heart attack

    c. Relief of severe pain

    d. Reduction of inflammation

43. A combination drug containing both pentazocine and naloxone would most likely be used to treat:

    a. Moderate to severe pain

    b. Seizures

    c. Symptoms of the common cold

    d. Hypertension

44. Which of the following is true regarding category D drugs?

    a. They may be safely used in pregnant patients.

    b. Animal studies indicate some risk, but the drug appears to be safe for humans.

    c. They should be used in pregnant patients only if the potential benefit justifies the potential risk to the fetus.

    d. They should not be used in pregnant patients under any circumstances.

45. Which of the following is used to treat seizures?

    a. Thiopental sodium (Pentothal)

    b. Fluoxetine (Prozac)

    c. Valproic acid (Depakote)

    d. Haloperidol (Haldol)

CASE STUDY APPLICATIONS

46. Mr. L, age 57, is an obese patient who has suffered two minor heart attacks in the past 3 years. Last year, his mitral valve was replaced. His blood pressure has been high for many years; however, it now appears to be controlled using various drugs. His LDL cholesterol was recently measured at 190 mg/dl and his triglycerides were 900 mg/dl. He does not smoke, and he walks 1/4 mile twice a week. He is taking the following medications:

    Aspirin
    Nifedipine (Procardia)
    Chlorothiazide (Diuril)

    a. What are the likely rationales for each of the drugs currently being taken by Mr. L?

    b. Does his clinical history warrant the addition of an antihyperlipidemic?

    c. Are there any lifestyle suggestions you might offer to Mr. L?

47. Ms. H, age 35, is about 25 pounds overweight. She exercises regularly and has been taking 40 mg/day of atorvastatin (Lipitor) for the past 2 years. Although her blood lipid profile was normal 12 months ago, her lipid levels have been gradually increasing. Her blood lipid levels are now in the high range.

    a. What are some possibilities as to why Ms. H's lipid levels have returned to higher than normal levels?

    b. What are some therapeutic options that might help these lipid levels return to normal?

CHAPTER 17

DRUGS FOR HYPERTENSION

LEARNING OUTCOMES

To view the objectives, please refer to the textbook or MyNursingKit™ at www.mynursingkit.com.

TRUE/FALSE

For Questions 1–6, choose T for true or F for false.

T F 1. The most common adverse effect of angiotensin-converting enzyme (ACE) inhibitors is dehydration.

T F 2. The death rate from cardiovascular-related diseases has dropped significantly over the past 20 years.

T F 3. Women in all ethnic groups experience more hypertension than men.

T F 4. Hypertension has a heredity component, with family members of hypertensives having a greater risk of this disease than nonfamily members.

T F 5. Alpha-adrenergic blockers lower blood pressure by dilating the smooth muscle in arterioles.

T F 6. The most common class of drugs used to treat hypertension is the direct-acting vasodilators.

FILL IN THE BLANK

From the text, find the correct word(s) to complete the statement(s).

7. The most common type of hypertension, accounting for 90% of all cases, is called _____.

8. As cardiac output increases, the blood pressure _____.

9. Angiotensin II raises blood pressure by _____.

10. Calcium channel blockers cause the smooth muscle in arterioles to _____, thus _____ blood pressure.

 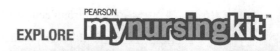

11. ACE inhibitors, such as captopril (Capoten), reduce blood pressure by lowering levels of _____ and _____.

12. _____ is a condition that occurs when the heart rate increases due to the rapid fall in blood pressure created by a drug.

13. The adverse effects of adrenergic blockers are generally predictable, because they are usually extensions of the _____ response.

MATCHING

For Questions 14–23, match the drug in Column I with its pharmacologic classification in Column II.

Column I	Column II
14. _____ Clonidine (Catapres)	a. Diuretic
15. _____ Captopril (Capoten)	b. Calcium channel blocker
16. _____ Spironolactone (Aldactone)	c. ACE inhibitor or angiotensin receptor blocker
17. _____ Diltiazem (Cardizem)	d. Beta$_1$-blocker
18. _____ Losartan (Cozaar)	e. Alpha$_1$-blocker
19. _____ Verapamil (Calan)	f. Centrally acting alpha$_2$-adrenergic agent
20. _____ Lisinopril (Prinivil, Zestril)	g. Direct vasodilator
21. _____ Hydralazine (Apresoline)	
22. _____ Metoprolol (Toprol)	
23. _____ Hydrochlorothiazide (Microzide)	

MULTIPLE CHOICE

24. Which of the following lowers blood pressure primarily by increasing the renal excretion of sodium and water?

    a. Doxazosin (Cardura)

    b. Furosemide (Lasix)

    c. Verapamil (Calan)

    d. Quinapril (Accupril)

25. Which of the following is a cardioselective beta$_1$-blocker?

    a. Propranolol (Inderal)

    b. Doxazosin (Cardura)

    c. Ipratropium (Atrovent)

    d. Atenolol (Tenormin)

26. A blood pressure of 138/83 mmHg in a patient over 80 years old with no compelling indications would be considered:

    a. A reason to begin diuretic therapy

    b. A reason to begin aggressive therapy with furosemide (Lasix)

    c. Normal

    d. A reason to begin therapy with sympatholytics

27. All of the following are primary factors responsible for blood pressure EXCEPT:

    a. Venous pressure

    b. Cardiac output

    c. Resistance of the small arteries

    d. Blood volume

28. As it relates to antihypertensive therapy, stepped care is:

    a. Two or more drugs from the same class

    b. Two or more drugs from different classes

    c. One drug during weeks 1–3, then a new drug starting in week 4

    d. 1 week of drug therapy alternating with 1 week of no drug administration

29. Which drug class is NOT commonly used to treat hypertension?

    a. Calcium channel blockers

    b. ACE inhibitors

    c. Direct-acting vasodilators

    d. Sodium channel blockers

30. Which drug class contains first-choice drugs for treating mild to moderate hypertension because they act on the kidney tubule to block reabsorption of sodium?

    a. Diuretics

    b. Calcium channel blockers

    c. Direct vasodilators

    d. Alpha blockers

31. When assessing laboratory tests, the health care provider should know that hyperkalemia is a common adverse effect of therapy with:

    a. Diuretics

    b. Calcium channel blockers

    c. Direct vasodilators

    d. Alpha blockers

32. Calcium channel blockers used for hypertension act by blocking calcium ion channels in:

    a. Skeletal muscle

    b. Vascular smooth muscle

    c. The central nervous system (CNS)

    d. The kidney

33. Which drug class inhibits the secretion of aldosterone?

    a. Diuretics

    b. Calcium channel blockers

    c. ACE inhibitors

    d. Alpha blockers

34. Which of the following drug classes are used to treat hypertension?

    a. Sympathomimetics

    b. Selective $beta_1$-blockers

    c. Selective $beta_2$-blockers

    d. Parasympathomimetics

35. When assessing the patient, the health care provider should know that bradycardia is a common adverse effect with:

    a. Selective $beta_1$-blockers

    b. Calcium channel blockers

    c. ACE inhibitors

    d. Alpha blockers

36. Which of the following drugs would be prescribed on an emergency basis to lower extremely high blood pressure within minutes?

    a. Hydralazine (Apresoline)

    b. Nitroprusside (Nitropress)

    c. Doxazosin (Cardura)

    d. Prazosin (Minipress)

37. In response to falling blood pressure, the kidney releases:

    a. Renin

    b. Aldosterone

    c. Angiotensin

    d. Potassium

38. The health care provider should use caution when administering which class of antihypertensives to patients with asthma due to possible bronchoconstriction?

    a. Alpha blockers

    b. Calcium channel blockers

    c. ACE inhibitors

    d. Beta blockers

DO YOU REMEMBER?

39. Which of the following should be taken 1–2 hours before other drugs because it may bind to other medications?

    a. Cholestyramine (Questran)

    b. Atorvastatin (Lipitor)

    c. Niacin

    d. Morphine

40. Which of the following routes for hydromorphone would the nurse use to achieve the most rapid onset of action?

    a. PO 8 mg

    b. Subcutaneous 1.5 mg

    c. IV 0.80 mg

    d. Rectal 3 mg

41. For hypertension, an average daily dose is 5 mg for enalapril and 10 mg for fosinopril. From this information, you may correctly conclude that:

    a. Enalapril is twice as effective as fosinopril.

    b. Enalapril will likely produce fewer side effects than fosinopril.

    c. Enalapril is more potent than fosinopril.

    d. The onset of action for fosinopril will be longer than that of enalapril.

42. Atropine is a prototype for which drug class?

    a. Sympathomimetics

    b. Beta-adrenergic blockers

    c. Parasympathomimetics

    d. Cholinergic blockers

43. Which of the following drugs is often combined in cartridges with local anesthetics?

    a. Epinephrine

    b. Atropine

    c. Heparin

    d. Acetaminophen

CASE STUDY APPLICATIONS

44. Mr. H, age 50, has presented a blood pressure of 170/100 mmHg the last three visits to his doctor. Hydrochlorothiazide (Microzide) was prescribed for him about 1 year ago. Other than some anxiety, he offers no complaints and other vital signs are normal. His blood lipids are elevated, he is 20 pounds overweight, and he smokes one pack of cigarettes a day; otherwise, he appears healthy.

    a. What nonpharmacologic therapies would you recommend for Mr. H?

    b. You suspect that Mr. H has not been taking his medication. How would you convince him to take his medication, despite the fact that he feels fine?

    c. Assuming that he has been taking his medication, what is the next logical pharmacologic option for Mr. H?

45. Ms. F is a 75-year-old woman who has been taking enalapril (Vasotec) and chlorothiazide for hypertension for the past 2 years. She is very compliant, taking walks daily, watching her salt intake, and eating plenty of potassium-rich foods such as bananas. Two weeks ago, her physician increased her dose of enalapril and switched her to spironolactone instead of chlorothiazide. She is now in the office complaining that she gets dizzy and falls over every morning when she gets out of bed, and she feels like her heart is racing when she walks. Although her blood pressure is normal, Ms. F wants to be switched back to her previous medications.

    a. What might be the cause of her dizziness? What teaching might be done to help solve this problem?

    b. An electrocardiogram (ECG) on Ms. F is normal. Can you recognize anything in her history that might be responsible for her heart complaints? What questions would you ask to better define her problem?

    c. Is it necessary to change Ms. F's medication, or might her complaints be resolved through patient teaching?

46. A patient has been receiving nicardipine (Cardene) for hypertension for 6 months and blood pressure has been brought to within normal values. Propranolol, a drug that decreases the hepatic metabolism of nicardipine, is added to treat the patient's angina.

    a. How would you predict that this effect on metabolism would change the effectiveness of nicardipine?

    b. Both of these drugs affect the heart. Would you expect their effects to be additive or antagonistic? What cardiac symptoms might the patient experience?

    c. When propranolol is added, how should the dose of nicardipine be adjusted?

CHAPTER 18

DRUGS FOR HEART FAILURE

LEARNING OUTCOMES

To view the objectives, please refer to the textbook or MyNursingKit™ at www.mynursingkit.com.

TRUE/FALSE

For Questions 1–5, choose T for true or F for false.

T F 1. Medications are available that have the potential to cure heart failure (HF) in a large percentage of patients.

T F 2. In healthy patients, the amount of blood received by the right side of the heart is less than that sent out by the left side.

T F 3. Left HF is also called congestive HF.

T F 4. HF may occur on the right side, left side, or both sides of the heart.

T F 5. Direct vasodilators have become first-choice drugs in the treatment of HF.

 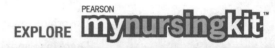
FILL IN THE BLANK

From the text, find the correct word(s) to complete the statement(s).

6. A slower heart rate provides a longer time for the myocardium to rest between beats, thus decreasing the _____ on the heart.

7. As more stretch is applied to myocardial fibers, they will contract with _____ force.

8. As a general rule, if the heart rate is less than _____ beats per minute, digoxin (Lanoxin) should be withheld.

MATCHING

For Questions 9–19, match the drug in Column I with its classification in Column II.

Column I

9. _____ Lisinopril (Prinivil)

10. _____ Hydralazine (Apresoline)

11. _____ Carvedilol (Coreg)

12. _____ Hydrochlorothiazide (Microzide)

13. _____ Milrinone (Primacor)

14. _____ Amrinone (Inocor)

15. _____ Quinapril (Accupril)

16. _____ Triamterene (Dyrenium)

17. _____ Enalapril (Vasotec)

18. _____ Isosorbide dinitrate (Isordil)

19. _____ Digoxin (Lanoxin)

Column II

a. Diuretic

b. Cardiac glycoside

c. Angiotensin-converting enzyme (ACE) inhibitor

d. Beta blocker

e. Direct vasodilator

f. Phosphodiesterase inhibitor

MULTIPLE CHOICE

20. The primary action of digoxin (Lanoxin) that makes it effective in treating HF is its ability to:

    a. Dilate the coronary arteries

    b. Increase impulse conduction across the myocardium

    c. Decrease blood pressure

    d. Increase cardiac contractility/output

21. It is critical for the nurse to evaluate blood electrolyte levels during digoxin therapy. Which of the following will significantly reduce the effectiveness of digoxin?

    a. Hypokalemia

    b. Hyperkalemia

    c. Hypocalcemia

    d. Hypercalcemia

22. HF is best defined as:

    a. Enlargement of the heart

    b. Inability of the heart to beat in a coordinated manner

    c. Inability of the ventricles to pump sufficient blood

    d. Congestion in the lungs caused by damage to the myocardium

23. The amount of blood pumped per minute by each ventricle is the:

    a. Preload

    b. Afterload

    c. Stroke volume

    d. Cardiac output

24. Preload is defined as the:

    a. Amount of blood pumped per minute by each ventricle

    b. Degree to which the heart fibers are stretched just prior to contraction

    c. Pressure in the aorta that must be overcome for blood to be ejected from the heart

    d. Ability to increase the strength of contraction

25. Which of the following drug classes was first derived from the common plant known as the purple foxglove?

    a. Cardiac glycosides

    b. ACE inhibitors

    c. Phosphodiesterase inhibitors

    d. Beta-adrenergic blockers

26. Cardiac glycosides help the heart beat more forcefully:

    a. With a faster heart rate

    b. With a slower heart rate

    c. With no effect on cardiac output

    d. With a diminished cardiac output

27. Digoxin (Lanoxin) acts by:

    a. Blocking beta-adrenergic receptors in the heart

    b. Stimulating beta-adrenergic receptors in the heart

    c. Inhibiting Na^+–K^+ ATPase

    d. Stimulating Na^+–K^+ ATPase

28. Which of the following is NOT a beneficial action of digoxin in a patient with HF?

    a. Increased heart rate

    b. Increased cardiac output

    c. Increased urine production

    d. Decreased peripheral edema

29. During digoxin therapy, the nurse must monitor for which serious adverse effect?

    a. Permanent visual disturbances

    b. Hyperkalemia

    c. Hypotension

    d. Dysrhythmias

30. Which drug class has replaced the cardiac glycosides as first-choice drugs in the therapy of HF?

    a. Direct vasodilators

    b. ACE inhibitors

    c. Phosphodiesterase inhibitors

    d. Beta-adrenergic blockers

31. The primary action of the ACE inhibitors that benefits a patient with HF is a decrease in:

    a. Peripheral resistance/blood pressure

    b. Cardiac output

    c. Heart rate

    d. Urine output

32. By what mechanism does isosorbide dinitrate (Isordil) benefit patients with HF?

    a. Lowering arterial blood pressure

    b. Increasing urine output

    c. Reducing venous return, causing a decrease in cardiac workload

    d. Slowing the heart rate, causing a reduction in cardiac workload

33. In addition to HF, hydralazine (Apresoline) is also prescribed for:

    a. Coagulation disorders

    b. Hypertension

    c. Stroke

    d. Glaucoma

34. In addition to HF, diuretics are also commonly prescribed for:

    a. Minor depression

    b. Coagulation disorders

    c. Hypertension

    d. Dysrhythmias

35. By what mechanism do diuretics, such as furosemide (Lasix), improve the symptoms of patients with HF?

    a. Blockading beta-adrenergic receptors

    b. Causing the heart to beat with more strength

    c. Reducing fluid/plasma volume

    d. Slowing heart rate, thus reducing cardiac workload

36. During furosemide therapy, the health care provider must monitor for which serious adverse effect?

    a. Electrolyte imbalances

    b. Dysrhythmias

    c. Reflex tachycardia

    d. Hypertension

37. The primary use of the phosphodiesterase inhibitors in patients with HF is to:

    a. Cause a rapid reduction in fluid/plasma volume

    b. Cause the heart to beat faster

    c. Rapidly lower blood pressure

    d. Increase the force of contraction and increase cardiac output

38. Beta-adrenergic blockers, such as carvedilol (Coreg), may improve HF by:

    a. Increasing the heart rate

    b. Decreasing the heart rate

    c. Causing the heart to contract with more force

    d. Lowering blood pressure and reducing cardiac workload

DO YOU REMEMBER?

39. Which of the following classes of drugs is NOT prescribed for hypertension?

    a. Sodium channel blockers

    b. ACE inhibitors

    c. Beta blockers

    d. Diuretics

40. Patients are often advised to eat plenty of bananas during drug therapy with the thiazide diuretics in order to get a sufficient supply of:

    a. Selenium

    b. Calcium

    c. Potassium

    d. Chloride

41. A typical dose of carvedilol is 6.25 mg bid. The term *bid* means:

    a. Twice a week

    b. Twice a day

    c. Before bedtime

    d. Before breakfast

42. Which of the following is NOT a drug class that has significant potential for abuse by patients?

    a. Barbiturates

    b. Benzodiazepines

    c. Opioids

    d. Triptans

43. Which class may be used to dry secretions, treat asthma, and prevent motion sickness?

    a. Anticholinergics

    b. Cholinergics

    c. Parasympathomimetics

    d. Alpha blockers

CASE STUDY APPLICATIONS

44. Drugs can affect the heart in a number of ways. It is essential that the health care provider understand the underlying cardiac pathophysiology in order to predict drug action.

    a. Explain the difference between an inotropic effect and a chronotropic effect.

    b. Give examples of pharmacologic classes of drugs that affect each.

    c. In general, is it more desirable to give a drug with a positive inotropic effect or a positive chronotropic effect when treating a patient with chronic HF? Explain your answer.

45. Mr. L has just been diagnosed with early HF and his physician has prescribed hydrochlorothiazide (Microzide), atorvastatin (Lipitor), and lisinopril (Prinivil). His blood pressure is slightly elevated, his blood cholesterol is marginally high, and he has stenosis of the mitral valve, which seems to be worsening. Although not an athletic person, Mr. L. likes to take long walks after dinner. He confides that, at his age of 60, he has no intention of taking any of the medications but intends to try Chinese herbal therapy.

    a. What is the rationale for each of the medications?

    b. What would be your advice to Mr. L regarding his decision not to take the prescription medications?

    c. What lifestyle changes would you suggest to Mr. L to improve his cardiac health?

CHAPTER 19

DRUGS FOR DYSRHYTHMIAS

LEARNING OUTCOMES

To view the objectives, please refer to the textbook or MyNursingKit™ at www.mynursingkit.com.

TRUE/FALSE

For Questions 1–6, choose T for true or F for false.

T F 1. Most dysrhythmias are life threatening and require immediate treatment.

T F 2. Dysrhythmias that originate in the ventricles are generally more serious, because they more often interfere with the normal function of the heart.

T F 3. Under resting conditions, Na^+ and Ca^{2+} are found in higher concentrations *inside* myocardial cells, whereas K^+ is found in higher concentration *outside* these cells.

T F 4. Digoxin should never be administered to a patient diagnosed with dysrhythmias.

T F 5. Dysrhythmias are often associated with other diseases, such as hypertension and heart failure.

T F 6. Antidysrhythmic agents have the ability to cause rhythm abnormalities or worsen existing ones.

FILL IN THE BLANK

From the text, find the correct word(s) to complete the statement(s).

7. After the action potential has passed, repolarization of the myocardial cell depends on removal of _____ from the cell.

8. Calcium channel blockers are most effective against _____ dysrhythmias.

9. Label the parts of the conduction pathway and the events of the electrocardiogram (ECG) in the figure below.

A. _____

B. _____

C. _____

D. _____

E. _____

F. _____

G. _____

H. _____

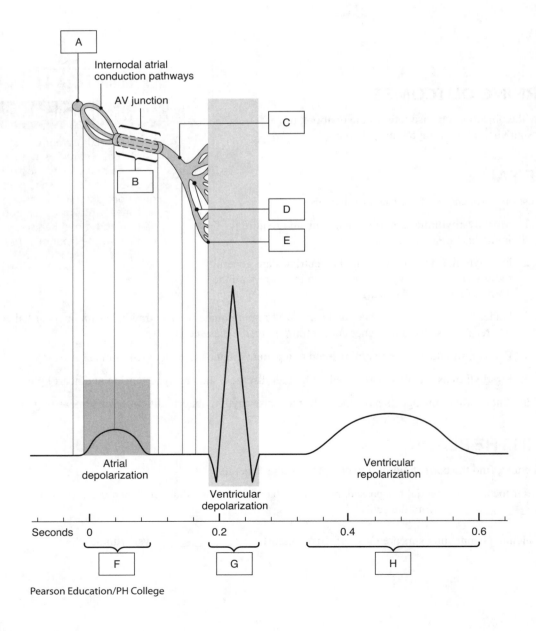

Pearson Education/PH College

MATCHING

For Questions 10–21, match the drug in Column I with its classification in Column II.

Column I	Column II
10. _____ Quinidine sulfate (Quinidex)	a. Sodium channel blocker
11. _____ Esmolol (Brevibloc)	b. Potassium channel blocker
12. _____ Amiodarone (Cordarone)	c. Beta-adrenergic blocker
13. _____ Diltiazem (Cardizem)	d. Calcium channel blocker
14. _____ Ibutilide (Corvert)	e. Miscellaneous (none of the above)
15. _____ Verapamil (Calan)	
16. _____ Phenytoin (Dilantin)	
17. _____ Lidocaine (Xylocaine)	
18. _____ Sotalol (Betapace)	
19. _____ Procainamide (Procanbid)	
20. _____ Adenosine (Adenocard)	
21. _____ Disopyramide (Norpace)	

MULTIPLE CHOICE

22. Dysrhythmias are best described as:

    a. Abnormalities of electrical conduction in the heart

    b. Diminished cardiac output

    c. Narrowing of the coronary arteries

    d. High blood pressure

23. Which of the following is NOT a type of dysrhythmia?

    a. Atrial tachycardia

    b. Ventricular flutter

    c. Sinus bradycardia

    d. Premature subventricular contractions

24. Electrical impulses in the heart generally begin in the:

    a. Atrioventricular bundle

    b. Atrioventricular (AV) node

    c. Sinoatrial (SA) node

    d. Purkinje fibers

25. In most myocardial cells and in neurons, an action potential begins when channels located in the plasma membrane open and _____ rushes into the cell, producing a rapid depolarization.

    a. Calcium

    b. Phosphate

    c. Potassium

    d. Sodium

26. Which of the following is NOT a class of drugs for treating dysrhythmias?

    a. Sodium channel blockers

    b. Alpha-adrenergic blockers

    c. Potassium channel blockers

    d. Calcium channel blockers

27. The basic mechanism by which nearly all antidysrhythmic drugs act to terminate or prevent abnormal rhythms is to:

    a. Increase heart rate until the rhythm returns to normal

    b. Dilate the coronary arteries, so that more blood gets to the myocardium

    c. Slow the impulse conduction velocity until the rhythm returns to normal

    d. Decrease blood pressure, so that the heart has less workload

28. A blockade of sodium channels in myocardial cells will:

    a. Slow the spread of impulse conduction

    b. Speed up the spread of impulse conduction

    c. Stop the spread of impulse conduction

    d. Worsen a dysrhythmia

29. Lidocaine is given _____ to terminate _____ dysrhythmias.

    a. PO, ventricular

    b. PO, atria

    c. IV, atrial

    d. IV, ventricular

30. Which antidysrhythmic drug acts by blocking beta-adrenergic receptors in the heart?

    a. Verapamil (Calan)

    b. Digoxin (Lanoxin)

    c. Amiodarone (Cordarone)

    d. Propranolol (Inderal)

31. Which of the following is the sodium channel blocker that is the oldest antidysrhythmic drug?

    a. Propranolol (Inderal)

    b. Amiodarone (Cordarone)

    c. Quinidine sulfate (Quinidex)

    d. Verapamil (Calan)

32. The nurse is administering procainamide (Procanbid) for acute tachycardia. The nurse will assess for which unusual drug adverse effect that can affect 30–50% of patients?

    a. Stevens-Johnson syndrome

    b. Lupus

    c. Lymphoma

    d. Aplastic anemia

33. Beta-adrenergic blockers are used to treat a large number of cardiovascular diseases. Which of the following is NOT one of the uses of beta blockers?

    a. Anticoagulant

    b. Hypertension

    c. Heart failure

    d. Dysrhythmias

34. The way that beta-adrenergic blockers prevent dysrhythmias is to:

    a. Speed up impulse conduction across the myocardium

    b. Slow impulse conduction across the myocardium

    c. Blockade calcium channels

    d. Blockade sodium channels

35. Propranolol (Inderal) is classified as a:

    a. Nonselective alpha and beta blocker

    b. Nonselective beta blocker

    c. Selective $beta_1$-blocker

    d. Selective $beta_2$-blocker

36. Which of the following is NOT an expected adverse effect in a patient taking propranolol (Inderal)?

    a. Diminished sex drive

    b. Hypotension

    c. Bradycardia

    d. Tachycardia

37. Potassium channel blockers prevent dysrhythmias by:

    a. Blocking beta-adrenergic receptors in the myocardium

    b. Reducing blood pressure

    c. Interfering with calcium ion channels

    d. Prolonging the refractory period of the heart

38. Which potassium channel blocker has become a preferred drug for the treatment of atrial dysrhythmias in patients with heart failure?

    a. Ibutilide (Corvert)

    b. Dofetilide (Tikosyn)

    c. Amiodarone (Cordarone)

    d. Sotalol (Betapace)

39. During amiodarone (Cordarone) therapy, the nurse should monitor for serious adverse effects related to which body system?

    a. Central nervous system (CNS)

    b. Pulmonary

    c. Cardiovascular

    d. Gastrointestinal

40. Blocking calcium ion channels has a number of effects on the heart and vascular system. These effects are most similar to those of:

    a. Sodium channel blockers

    b. Potassium channel blockers

    c. Beta-adrenergic blockers

    d. Cardiac glycosides

41. Which of the following antidysrhythmics would the health care provider administer intravenously to rapidly terminate serious atrial dysrhythmias?

    a. Adenosine (Adenocard)

    b. Amiodarone (Cordarone)

    c. Propranolol (Inderal)

    d. Verapamil (Calan)

DO YOU REMEMBER?

42. The primary indication for phosphodiesterase inhibitors is:

    a. Hypertension

    b. Coagulation disorders

    c. Heart failure

    d. Shock

43. In addition to its use in treating dysrhythmias, lidocaine is widely used as a(n):

    a. Local anesthetic

    b. Antihypertensive

    c. Antimigraine agent

    d. General anesthetic

44. Which of the following is the most widely used drug class for the treatment of depression?

    a. Barbiturates

    b. Na^+-K^+ ATPase inhibitors

    c. Benzodiazepines

    d. Selective serotonin reuptake inhibitors

45. A patient taking sumatriptan (Imitrex) likely suffers from:

    a. Sleep disorders

    b. Seizures

    c. Migraines

    d. Schizophrenia

46. Gamma aminobutyric acid (GABA) is a:

    a. Surgical procedure used to help patients with psychosis

    b. Neurotransmitter

    c. Drug used to treat bipolar disorder

    d. Widely abused hallucinogen

CASE STUDY APPLICATIONS

47. Ms. D, 67 years old, is brought to the hospital by paramedics after collapsing on the street. She has a history of heart failure and has been taking digoxin and furosemide. The emergency department (ED) physician determines that she is experiencing a myocardial infarction accompanied by a severe ventricular dysrhythmia. Her blood pressure is normal but her heart rate is only 45. The following drugs were among those administered during her 5-day hospital stay:

    Lidocaine (in the ER)
    Aspirin
    Hydromorphone (Dilaudid)

    a. What is the rationale for each of the drugs?

    b. Why would a beta blocker likely be contraindicated for Ms. D?

    c. Can you offer a pharmacologic explanation for Ms. D's initial symptoms?

48. Some cardiac drugs may benefit multiple disorders. What classes of drugs might be prescribed for patients who have both dysrhythmia and the following?

    a. Heart failure

    b. Hypertension

    c. Migraines

    d. Seizures

CHAPTER 20

DRUGS FOR COAGULATION DISORDERS

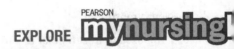

LEARNING OUTCOMES

To view the objectives, please refer to the textbook or MyNursingKit™ at www.mynursingkit.com.

TRUE/FALSE

For Questions 1–5, choose T for true or F for false.

T   F   1. Because heparin is not absorbed by the gastrointestinal mucosa, the drug must be administered subcutaneously (SC) or through intravenous (IV) infusion.

T   F   2. Prothrombin time (PT) is a laboratory test often used to assess the effectiveness of warfarin (Coumadin) therapy.

T   F   3. Thrombolytics, such as alteplase (Activase), are used to dissolve thrombi.

T   F   4. Hemostasis is an abnormal process that often results in thrombi and emboli.

T   F   5. Regardless of the mechanism of drug action, all anticoagulant drugs decrease the normal time the body takes to form clots.

FILL IN THE BLANK

From the text, find the correct word(s) to complete the statement(s).

6. Fill in the blanks in the figure below.

   A. _____

   B. _____

   C. _____

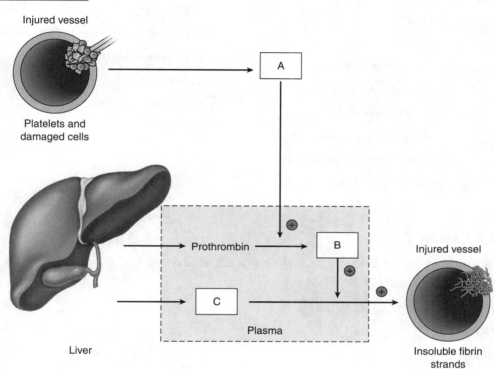

7. Fill in the blanks in the figure below.

   A. _____

   B. _____

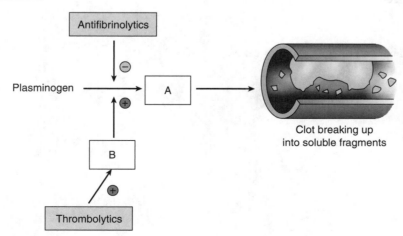

MATCHING

For Questions 8–18, match the drug in Column I with its classification in Column II.

Column I

8. _____ Warfarin (Coumadin)

9. _____ Abciximab (ReoPro)

10. _____ Dalteparin (Fragmin)

11. _____ Aspirin

12. _____ Aprotinin (Trasylol)

13. _____ Enoxaparin (Lovenox)

14. _____ Alteplase (Activase, tPA)

15. _____ Reteplase (Retavase)

16. _____ Tirofiban (Aggrastat)

17. _____ Aminocaproic acid (Amicar)

18. _____ Ticlopidine (Ticlid)

Column II

a. Anticoagulant: general type

b. Anticoagulant: antiplatelet type

c. Anticoagulant: low molecular weight heparin (LMWH) type

d. Adenosine diphosphate (ADP) receptor blocker

e. Glycoprotein IIb/IIIa blocker

f. Thrombolytic

g. Hemostatic (antifibrinolytic)

MULTIPLE CHOICE

19. The health care provider should never give aspirin to a patient who is taking:

    a. Streptokinase

    b. Warfarin (Coumadin)

    c. LMWHs

    d. Heparin

20. Which of the following clump and adhere to the wall of an injured blood vessel to begin the process of hemostasis?

    a. Platelets

    b. Red blood cells

    c. White blood cells

    d. Antibodies

21. The solid, insoluble part of a blood clot is called:

    a. Fibrin

    b. Thrombin

    c. Prothrombin

    d. Plasmin

22. Normal blood clotting occurs in about _____ minute(s).

    a. 1

    b. 3

    c. 6

    d. 10

23. Which organ is responsible for making many of the factors necessary for blood clotting?

    a. Kidney

    b. Liver

    c. Brain

    d. Skin

24. The process of clot removal is called:

    a. Embolysis

    b. Thrombolysis

    c. Plasminolysis

    d. Fibrinolysis

25. The specific class of drugs that promotes the formation of clots is called:

    a. Antifibrinolytics

    b. Thrombolytics

    c. Fibrinolytics

    d. Plasminogen activators

26. The health care provider should assess which laboratory test during therapy with heparin?

    a. Bleeding time

    b. Prothrombin time (PT)

    c. International normalized ratio (INR)

    d. Activated partial thromboplastin time (aPTT)

27. Anticoagulants are drugs that:

    a. Dissolve thrombi that have been recently formed

    b. Shorten PT time

    c. Prevent thrombi from forming or growing larger

    d. Cause platelets to become less sticky

28. What is the primary advantage of using LMWHs over heparin?

    a. LMWHs possess greater anticoagulant activity.

    b. LMWHs may be given by the oral route.

    c. LMWHs produce a more stable effect on coagulation; thus, fewer laboratory tests are needed.

    d. LMWHs have a prolonged duration of action.

29. What is the most serious adverse effect of anticoagulant therapy?

    a. Severe headache

    b. Abnormal hemorrhage

    c. Electrolyte depletion

    d. Cardiac arrhythmia

30. If serious hemorrhage occurs during heparin therapy, the nurse should administer:

    a. Protamine sulfate

    b. Vitamin K

    c. ADP

    d. Desmopressin (DDAVP)

31. Unlike heparin, the anticoagulant activity of warfarin can take several _____ to reach its maximum effect.

    a. Minutes

    b. Hours

    c. Days

    d. Weeks

32. Vitamin K is an antidote for an overdose with:

    a. Aspirin

    b. Heparin and LMWH

    c. Aminocaproic acid (Amicar)

    d. Warfarin (Coumadin)

33. On discontinuation of therapy, the pharmacologic activity of warfarin can take up to _____ to diminish.

    a. 10 minutes

    b. 10 hours

    c. 48 hours

    d. 10 days

34. Aspirin causes its anticoagulant effect by inhibiting:

    a. Plasminogen

    b. Prothrombin

    c. Thromboxane A_2

    d. Glycoprotein IIb/IIIa

35. Glycoprotein IIb/IIIa inhibitors act by blocking the final step in:

    a. Hemostasis

    b. Platelet aggregation

    c. The activation of plasminogen

    d. The formation of vitamin K

36. The primary action of streptokinase is to convert plasminogen to:

    a. Plasminogen activator

    b. Plasmin

    c. Fibrin

    d. Fibrinogen

37. The primary use of antifibrinolytics is to:

    a. Dissolve thrombi

    b. Reverse the effects of anticoagulants

    c. Prevent thrombi

    d. Prevent excessive bleeding following surgery

38. All of the following are used to prevent and treat excessive bleeding following surgical procedures EXCEPT:

    a. Warfarin (Coumadin)

    b. Abciximab (ReoPro)

    c. Aminocaproic acid (Amicar)

    d. Tranexamic acid (Cyklokapron)

39. Which of the following is NOT an indication for thrombolytic therapy?

    a. Acute myocardial infarction (MI)

    b. Postoperative bleeding

    c. Pulmonary embolism

    d. Deep vein thrombosis (DVT)

DO YOU REMEMBER?

40. A patient is receiving warfarin, which is 98% bound to plasma proteins. The antidepressant paroxetine (Paxil), which is 95% bound, is added to the patient's daily medications. If the paroxetine displaces warfarin from its binding sites, which of the following will most likely occur?

    a. Toxicity to warfarin

    b. Toxicity to paroxetine

    c. Diminished effect from warfarin

    d. Diminished effect from paroxetine

41. The antidepressant imipramine (Tofranil) is metabolized to its active form, desipramine, in the liver. How should the dose of imipramine be adjusted for patients with liver cirrhosis?

    a. The dose should be increased above average.

    b. The dose should be decreased below average.

    c. An average dose should be used.

    d. These patients should not receive imipramine.

42. Which of the following is a widely used class of antipsychotic medication?

    a. Phenothiazines

    b. Benzodiazepines

    c. Monoamine oxidase (MAO) inhibitors

    d. Anticholinergics

43. The primary goal of the health care provider for pain management is to:

    a. Administer the least amount of pain medication possible

    b. Administer analgesics only when pain becomes intolerable

    c. Ensure that dependence does not develop

    d. Alleviate the pain

44. Of the following four drugs, which is NOT related to the other three?

    a. Phenytoin (Dilantin)

    b. Phenobarbital (Luminal)

    c. Sumatriptan (Imitrex)

    d. Ethosuximide (Zarontin)

CASE STUDY APPLICATIONS

45. Ms. S is being discharged from the hospital following surgery for replacement of a heart valve. She will be placed on warfarin (Coumadin) the remainder of her life due to the artificial valve.

    a. What activities would you suggest that Ms. S NOT perform due to her warfarin therapy?

    b. What types of signs or symptoms should Ms. S be taught to look for to avoid serious adverse effects from this drug?

    c. What medications would you advise Ms. S. to avoid should she experience headaches or joint pain?

46. Mr. P, a 50-year-old man, is being admitted to the hospital for the third time this year. He has a history of alcohol abuse, diabetes, and heart failure. Although he was brought in unconscious, the physician suspects a perforated ulcer with internal bleeding. The only medications that the paramedics found in Mr. P's house were a bottle of warfarin and a few packages of aspirin.

    a. What factors might have contributed to Mr. P's acute bleeding episode?

    b. How does Mr. P's history of alcohol abuse contribute to his condition?

    c. What medications might be ordered for Mr. P?

CHAPTER 21

DRUGS FOR ANGINA PECTORIS, MYOCARDIAL INFARCTION, AND CEREBROVASCULAR ACCIDENT

LEARNING OUTCOMES

To view the objectives, please refer to the textbook or MyNursingKit™ at www.mynursingkit.com.

TRUE/FALSE

For Questions 1–8, choose T for true or F for false.

T   F   1. A major goal of the health care provider is to determine the cause of chest pain quickly so that the proper treatment can be administered.

T   F   2. The myocardium receives most of its nutrients from the blood contained within the heart's chambers.

T   F   3. Physical and psychological dependence commonly occur with the long-acting organic nitrates if they are taken for extended periods.

T   F   4. Chest pain that does not respond following 3 doses of sublingual nitroglycerin may indicate that the patient is experiencing a stroke.

T   F   5. When treating a suspected myocardial infarction (MI), it is best to wait at least 8 hours after the onset of symptoms before administering anticoagulants.

T   F   6. Immediate treatment of stroke may reduce the degree of permanent disability caused by the disease.

T   F   7. Aspirin is usually contraindicated for patients at high risk for cerebrovascular accident.

T   F   8. Current drug therapy for stroke is largely a passive strategy involving waiting several days until the severity of the disease can be determined.

EXPLORE PEARSON 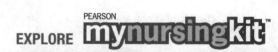 mynursingkit™

www.mynursingkit.com

MyNursingKit is your one stop for online chapter review materials and resources. Prepare for success with additional NCLEX®-style practice questions, interactive assignments and activities, web links, animations and videos, and more! Register your access code from the front of your book at www.mynursingkit.com.

FILL IN THE BLANK

From the text, find the correct word(s) to complete the statement(s).

9. Acute chest pain on physical exertion or emotional stress is characteristic of _____.

10. Atherosclerosis is due to a buildup of fatty, fibrous material, called _____, in the walls of arteries.

11. Drug therapy of stable angina is usually begun with _____.

12. Long-acting nitrates are often delivered through a(n) _____ to decrease the frequency and severity of anginal episodes.

13. An MI is the result of a sudden occlusion of a(n) _____.

14. After a clot in the coronary artery has been successfully dissolved, therapy with _____ is often initiated to prevent the formation of additional thrombi.

15. Stroke is caused by either a(n) _____ or _____ within a vessel serving the brain.

16. Drug therapy for thrombotic stroke focuses on two main goals: _____ and _____.

MATCHING

For Questions 17–26, match the drug in Column I with its classification in Column II.

Column I	Column II
17. _____ Lisinopril (Prinivil)	a. Organic nitrate
18. _____ Diltiazem (Cardizem)	b. Beta blocker
19. _____ Isosorbide dinitrate (Dilatrate SR)	c. Calcium channel blocker
20. _____ Metoprolol (Lopressor)	d. Angiotensin-converting enzyme (ACE) inhibitor
21. _____ Pentaerythrityl tetranitrate (Peritrate)	e. Analgesic
22. _____ Atenolol (Tenormin)	
23. _____ Nifedipine (Procardia)	
24. _____ Nitroglycerin (Nitrostat)	
25. _____ Timolol (Betimol)	
26. _____ Amlodipine (Norvasc)	

MULTIPLE CHOICE

27. Which of the following drug classes is used in the pharmacotherapy of angina pectoris?

    a. Calcium channel blockers

    b. ACE inhibitors

    c. HMG-CoA reductase inhibitors

    d. Cardiac glycosides

28. Which of the following best explains the mechanism by which organic nitrates terminate acute anginal attacks?

    a. Direct vasodilation of coronary arteries

    b. Slowing heart rate

    c. Stronger force of myocardial contraction

    d. Dilation of peripheral veins, reducing preload

29. The condition of having a reduced blood supply to myocardial cells is called:

    a. MI

    b. Angina pectoris

    c. Myocardial ischemia

    d. Stroke

30. Angina is most often preceded by:

    a. An aura

    b. Physical exertion or emotional excitement

    c. A sensation that the heart has skipped a beat

    d. Severe pain down the left arm

31. The pharmacologic goals for the treatment of angina are usually achieved by:

    a. Reducing cardiac workload

    b. Increasing the heart rate

    c. Increasing the force of myocardial contraction

    d. Increasing the amount of blood entering the heart

32. The vasodilation effect of organic nitrate agents is a result of the conversion of nitrate to the active form:

    a. Nitric oxide (NO)

    b. Nitrous oxide (N_2O)

    c. Nitroglycerin

    d. Hydrogen dioxide

33. By causing venodilation, nitrates reduce the amount of blood returning to the heart, thus decreasing:

    a. Heart rate

    b. Conduction velocity

    c. Blood pressure

    d. Cardiac output

34. In addition to causing venodilation, organic nitrates also have the ability to:

    a. Inhibit alpha$_1$-adrenergic receptors in arterioles

    b. Dilate the coronary arteries

    c. Terminate dysrhythmias

    d. Remove plaque from coronary arteries

35. Organic nitrates are classified based on whether they are:

    a. Parenteral or oral

    b. High or low potency

    c. Short or long acting

    d. Sedating or nonsedating

36. The nurse should administer which drug *sublingually* to terminate anginal pain?

    a. Atenolol (Tenormin)

    b. Diltiazem (Cardizem)

    c. Nitroglycerin (Nitro-Bid)

    d. Aspirin

37. The nurse should assess for which common adverse effect of nitroglycerin therapy?

    a. Headache

    b. Drowsiness

    c. Nausea/vomiting

    d. Hypotension

38. The primary mechanism by which beta-adrenergic blockers decrease the frequency of angina attacks is:

    a. Dilating the coronary arteries

    b. Increasing the heart rate

    c. Increasing the strength of contraction of the myocardium

    d. Reducing the cardiac workload

39. Which of the following is true regarding the effect of atenolol (Tenormin) on the heart?

    a. It selectively blocks $beta_1$-receptors.

    b. It nonselectively blocks $beta_1$- and $beta_2$-receptors.

    c. It selectively blocks $beta_2$-receptors.

    d. It has no effect on beta receptors.

40. The primary mechanism by which calcium channel blockers decrease the frequency of angina attacks is:

    a. Slowing conduction through the sinoatrial (SA) node

    b. Increasing the heart rate

    c. Increasing the strength of contraction of the myocardium

    d. Reducing cardiac workload

41. Calcium channel blockers are effective in treating variant angina because they:

    a. Lower blood pressure

    b. Slow the heart rate

    c. Slow conduction across the myocardium

    d. Relax arterial smooth muscle in the coronary arteries

42. Which of the following agents has the ability to inhibit the transport of calcium ions into myocardial cells and relaxes both coronary and peripheral blood vessels?

   a. Atenolol (Tenormin)

   b. Diltiazem (Cardizem)

   c. Nitroglycerin (Nitro-Bid)

   d. Reteplase (Retavase)

43. Which of the following is NOT a goal for the pharmacotherapy of acute MI?

   a. Restore blood supply to the damaged myocardium as quickly as possible

   b. Increase myocardial oxygen demand with organic nitrates or beta blockers

   c. Prevent associated dysrhythmias with antidysrhythmics

   d. Reduce post-MI mortality with aspirin and ACE inhibitors

44. In treating MI, the function of thrombolytic therapy is to:

   a. Restore blood supply to the damaged myocardium

   b. Decrease myocardial oxygen demand

   c. Control dysrhythmias

   d. Reduce acute pain associated with MI

45. The primary risk during thrombolytic therapy is:

   a. Hypertension

   b. Prolonged prothrombin time

   c. Excessive bleeding

   d. Dysrhythmia

46. Reteplase (Retavase) is most effective if administered not later than _____ after the onset of MI symptoms.

   a. 30 minutes

   b. 1 hour

   c. 6 hours

   d. 12 hours

47. Following an acute MI, metoprolol (Lopressor) is infused slowly until:

   a. The clot is dissolved

   b. Blood pressure falls to 100/70 mmHg

   c. A target heart rate of 60–90 beats per minute is reached

   d. The pain is relieved

48. Unless contraindicated, the nurse should administer 160 to 324 mg of aspirin as soon as possible following a suspected MI in order to:

    a. Restore blood supply to the damaged myocardium

    b. Decrease myocardial oxygen demand

    c. Reduce post-MI mortality

    d. Reduce acute pain associated with MI

49. Captopril (Capoten) and lisinopril (Prinivil) are sometimes administered to patients with MI to:

    a. Restore blood supply to the damaged myocardium

    b. Increase myocardial oxygen demand

    c. Reduce post-MI mortality

    d. Reduce acute pain associated with MI

50. Opioids, such as morphine sulfate, are sometimes administered to patients with MI to:

    a. Restore blood supply to the damaged myocardium

    b. Decrease myocardial oxygen demand

    c. Reduce post-MI mortality

    d. Reduce acute pain associated with MI

51. Patients at high risk for stroke are often treated with:

    a. Antidysrhythmics

    b. Antihypertensives

    c. Opioids

    d. Cardiac glycosides

DO YOU REMEMBER?

52. In addition to angina, organic nitrates are indicated for:

    a. Dysrhythmias

    b. Coagulation disorders

    c. Hypertension

    d. Heart failure

53. Nitrous oxide is classified as a(n):

    a. IV anesthetic

    b. Gas

    c. Volatile agent

    d. Local anesthetic

54. Extrapyramidal adverse effects are observed during therapy with which drug group?

    a. Antianxiety drugs

    b. Antipsychotics

    c. Antiepilepsy drugs

    d. Opioids

55. A patient taking lithium (Eskalith) is likely being treated for which of the following conditions?

    a. Bipolar disorder

    b. Schizophrenia

    c. Attention-deficit hyperactivity disorder

    d. Mild to moderate pain

56. A drug that blocks impulses from the parasympathetic nervous system is known as a:

    a. Sympathomimetic

    b. Beta-adrenergic blocker

    c. Cholinergic blocker

    d. Calcium channel blocker

CASE STUDY APPLICATIONS

57. Mr. M is a 70-year-old, 280-pound African American man admitted through the emergency department for a possible stroke. He has partial paralysis on his left side and is unable to speak. His blood pressure is 190/110 and his computed tomography (CT) scan confirms a recent cerebrovascular accident (CVA). He is a lifetime tobacco user. While in the hospital, Mr. M was given reteplase (Retavase), furosemide (Lasix), and heparin. After release from the hospital, his medications were switched to hydrochlorothiazide (Microzide), diltiazem (Cardizem), and aspirin.

    a. Given the risk factors, what might have contributed to the stroke?

    b. Give the rationales for each of Mr. M's medications.

    c. From the types of medications that Mr. M was given, can you determine whether he suffered from a hemorrhagic stroke or a thrombotic stroke? Explain.

58. Ms. R is a 72-year-old home-bound patient. She is clinically obese and has been diagnosed with chronic heart failure, hypertension, and angina. She has been "watching" her diet and has cut her tobacco consumption to one-half pack per day but does not feel that she is capable of exercising. Her latest complaint is that the frequency and intensity of her anginal pain have increased over the past 3 months. Ms. R is quite nervous about the possibility of having a heart attack. Her medications are isosorbide dinitrate (sustained release tablets), nitroglycerin (as needed), and lisinopril.

    a. What is the rationale for each of Ms. R's medications?

    b. Are there lifestyle changes that you would suggest to increase her quality of life?

    c. What are some possible explanations for Ms. R's current complaint?

CHAPTER 22

DRUGS FOR SHOCK AND ANAPHYLAXIS

LEARNING OUTCOMES

To view the objectives, please refer to the textbook or MyNursingKit™ at www.mynursingkit.com.

TRUE/FALSE

For Questions 1–3, choose T for true or F for false.

T   F   1. Most types of shock have a high mortality rate.

T   F   2. The adverse effects of dopamine may be quite serious due to the extremely long half-life of the drug.

T   F   3. Normal serum albumin is obtained from whole blood or plasma.

FILL IN THE BLANK

From the text, find the correct word(s) to complete the statement(s).

4. Shock is a clinical syndrome characterized by collapse of the _____ system.

5. The initial treatment of shock is often nonpharmacologic and includes the administration of _____.

6. In the early stages of shock, the body compensates for falling blood pressure by activating the _____ nervous system.

7. Norepinephrine (Levarterenol) acts directly on _____ adrenergic receptors to raise blood pressure.

8. Lactated Ringer's and normal saline are types of _____.

9. In addition to affecting the cardiovascular system, anaphylactic shock involves an abnormality in the _____ system.

10. An antigen may be defined as anything that is recognized as _____ by the immune system.

11. A fall in blood pressure sometimes causes a rebound speeding up of the heart known as _____.

MATCHING

For Questions 12–20, match the drug in Column I with its primary class in Column II.

Column I	Column II
12. _____ Norepinephrine (Levarterenol)	a. Vasoconstrictor/inotropic drug
13. _____ Fresh frozen plasma	b. Colloid
14. _____ Phenylephrine	c. Crystalloid
15. _____ Dextran 40	d. Blood product
16. _____ Normal saline	
17. _____ Dopamine (Dopastat, Intropin)	
18. _____ Hetastarch	
19. _____ 5% Dextrose in water	
20. _____ Dobutamine (Dobutrex)	

MULTIPLE CHOICE

21. If a patient receives a suspected overdose of epinephrine, the nurse must immediately assess for:

    a. Hypoglycemia

    b. Hypertension

    c. Bronchospasm

    d. Diarrhea

22. Shock is a condition characterized by:

    a. Extremely high blood pressure

    b. Abnormal cardiac rhythm

    c. Vital tissues not receiving enough blood to function properly

    d. The heart not pumping with sufficient contractility

23. Which of the following is NOT a common sign or symptom of shock?

    a. Weakness, without any specific symptoms

    b. Restlessness, anxiety, confusion, and lack of interest

    c. Thirst

    d. Hypertension

24. A weak or unresponsive patient with obvious trauma or bleeding to a limb might be experiencing _____ shock.

    a. Hypovolemic

    b. Neurogenic

    c. Cardiogenic

    d. Anaphylactic

25. In many types of shock, the nurse must recognize that the most serious medical challenge facing the patient is:

    a. Heart failure

    b. Brain damage

    c. Hypotension

    d. Myocardial infarction (MI)

26. The health care provider administers vasoconstrictors to patients with shock in order to:

    a. Prevent dysrhythmias

    b. Stabilize blood pressure

    c. Prevent postshock mortality

    d. Prevent blood pressure from rising to harmful levels

27. Most of the drugs used to raise blood pressure in patients with shock:

    a. Are central nervous system (CNS) stimulants

    b. Are CNS depressants

    c. Activate the parasympathetic nervous system

    d. Activate the sympathetic nervous system

28. Norepinephrine (Levarterenol) activates _____ adrenergic receptors.

    a. Alpha

    b. Beta$_1$

    c. Both alpha and beta$_1$

    d. Neither alpha nor beta$_1$

29. In addition to its use in shock, norepinephrine is indicated for:

    a. Cardiac arrest

    b. Hypertension

    c. Dysrhythmias

    d. Strokes

30. The primary use of inotropic drugs in the treatment of shock is to increase:

    a. Blood pressure

    b. The force of myocardial contraction

    c. Heart rate

    d. Conduction velocity across the myocardium

31. Dobutamine (Dobutrex) is a _____ that has value in the treatment of certain types of shock, due to its ability to cause the heart to beat more forcefully, without causing major effects on heart rate.

    a. Selective $beta_1$-blocker

    b. Cholinergic blocker

    c. Cardiac glycoside

    d. $Beta_1$-adrenergic agent

32. Dopamine (Intropin) is the immediate metabolic precursor to:

    a. Acetylcholine

    b. Norepinephrine

    c. Gamma-aminobutyric acid (GABA)

    d. Serotonin

33. During anaphylaxis, the body responds quickly by releasing massive amounts of:

    a. Prostaglandin

    b. Acetylcholinesterase

    c. Histamine

    d. Antihistamine

34. Which of the following would the nurse LEAST likely give to a patient experiencing anaphylactic shock?

    a. Morphine sulfate

    b. Oxygen

    c. Diphenhydramine (Benadryl)

    d. Albuterol (Proventil)

35. Epinephrine (Adrenalin) activates _____ adrenergic receptors.

    a. Alpha

    b. Beta

    c. Both alpha and beta

    d. Neither alpha nor beta

36. Within minutes after the nurse administers epinephrine (Adrenalin), activation of beta$_2$-adrenergic receptors will:

    a. Increase blood pressure

    b. Open the bronchi and relieve the patient's shortness of breath

    c. Stimulate the heart to beat more forcefully

    d. Relieve symptoms of hives and itching

37. A widespread inflammatory response to bacterial, fungal, or parasitic infection can result in which type of shock?

    a. Cardiogenic

    b. Hypovolemic

    c. Neurogenic

    d. Septic

DO YOU REMEMBER?

38. After administering a beta-adrenergic blocker, the health care provider should monitor the patient for which expected effect?

    a. Increased heart rate

    b. Lowered blood pressure

    c. Dilation of bronchial smooth muscle

    d. Increased myocardial contractility

39. Which of the following is a cholinergic blocker?

    a. Metoprolol (Lopressor)

    b. Succinylcholine (Anectine)

    c. Neostigmine (Prostigmin)

    d. Atropine sulfate

40. Which of the following is NOT classified as a nonsteroidal anti-inflammatory drug (NSAID)?

    a. Acetaminophen

    b. Aspirin

    c. Celecoxib (Celebrex)

    d. Ibuprofen

41. Antiplatelet agents are primarily prescribed to:

    a. Lower blood cholesterol

    b. Dissolve thrombi

    c. Prevent thromboembolic disease

    d. Prevent migraines

42. Most barbiturate use in children is limited to the treatment of:

    a. Sleep disorders

    b. Seizure disorders

    c. Depression

    d. Anxiety

CASE STUDY APPLICATIONS

43. Paramedics arrive at the scene of an automobile accident and discover Mr. V, a 35-year-old, who is wandering around the scene, confused. He has several superficial wounds that are bleeding, although the amount of blood loss does not appear to be great. Initial vital signs show slightly elevated blood pressure and heart rate with a weak pulse. The paramedics treat Mr. V's wounds, administer oxygen, and keep him warm and lying on a stretcher while they treat other injured people. Twenty minutes later, Mr. V is unresponsive with a blood pressure of 70/40 and no identifiable pulse. An electrocardiogram (ECG) reveals a ventricular dysrhythmia that appears to be quickly worsening. The paramedics immediately administer the following drugs:

    Dextran 70 (Macrodex)
    Norepinephrine (Levophed)
    Dobutamine (Dobutrex)
    Lidocaine (Xylocaine)

    a. Did the paramedics make an error in leaving Mr. V while they treated other patients? Defend your answer.

    b. Why did the patient not show serious signs of shock when the paramedics arrived?

    c. What is the therapeutic rationale for each of the drugs administered?

44. At the same automobile accident described in Question 43, paramedics find Ms. F, an elderly patient who obviously has hit her head on the windshield. She is unconscious and does not have other apparent trauma. Other than a few minor scrapes, no bleeding is evident. Vital signs show slow respirations, very low pulse rate, and a blood pressure of 94/52. Pupils are unresponsive to light.

    a. What type of shock is Ms. F most likely experiencing? What clues led you to this conclusion?

    b. What type of drugs would be helpful to reverse the symptoms of shock?

    c. What other supportive measures might be necessary?

CHAPTER 23

DIURETICS AND DRUGS FOR ELECTROLYTE AND ACID-BASE DISORDERS

LEARNING OUTCOMES

To view the objectives, please refer to the textbook or MyNursingKit™ at www.mynursingkit.com.

TRUE/FALSE

For Questions 1–4, choose T for true or F for false.

T   F   1. Patients with renal failure usually receive higher drug doses than normal.

T   F   2. Patients taking thiazide or loop diuretics are usually instructed to avoid food containing potassium.

T   F   3. When the body's pH drops below 7.35, acidosis occurs and symptoms of central nervous system (CNS) depression may be observed.

T   F   4. Increasing the renal excretion of bicarbonate ion will increase the acidity of the blood.

FILL IN THE BLANK

From the text, find the correct word(s) to complete the statement(s).

5. Thiazide diuretics act on the _____ tubule of the nephron.

6. When sodium reabsorption in the nephron is blocked, urine output will _____.

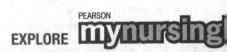

7. Identify the parts of the nephron shown in the figure below.

A. _____

B. _____

C. _____

D. _____

E. _____

F. _____

G. _____

H. _____

I. _____

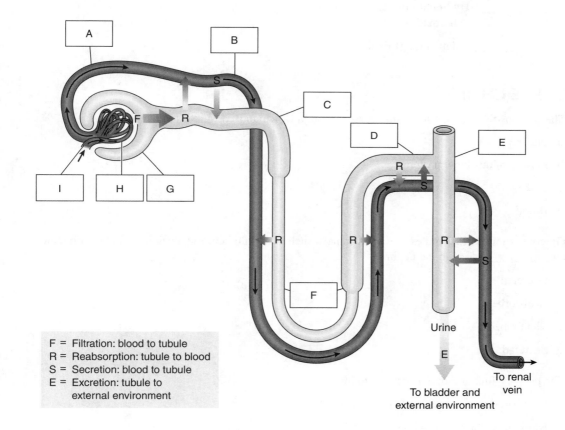

F = Filtration: blood to tubule
R = Reabsorption: tubule to blood
S = Secretion: blood to tubule
E = Excretion: tubule to
    external environment

MATCHING

For Questions 8–16, match the drug in Column I with its primary class in Column II.

Column I	Column II
8. _____ Bumetanide (Bumex)	a. Loop diuretic
9. _____ Triamterene (Dyrenium)	b. Thiazide or thiazide-like diuretic
10. _____ Metolazone (Zaroxolyn)	c. Potassium-sparing diuretic
11. _____ Mannitol (Osmitrol)	d. Carbonic anhydrase inhibitor diuretic
12. _____ Spironolactone (Aldactone)	e. Osmotic diuretic
13. _____ Acetazolamide (Diamox)	
14. _____ Furosemide (Lasix)	
15. _____ Hydrochlorothiazide (Microzide)	
16. _____ Indapamide (Lozol)	

MULTIPLE CHOICE

17. The composition of the filtrate that passes through Bowman's capsule is similar to that of:

    a. Plasma

    b. Plasma minus large proteins

    c. Urine

    d. Blood

18. Glucose, amino acids, and essential substances such as sodium, chloride, calcium, and bicarbonate are _____ in the nephron.

    a. Excreted

    b. Reabsorbed

    c. Metabolized

    d. Secreted

19. The primary function of a diuretic is to increase:

    a. Reabsorption of water in the nephron

    b. Blood flow through Bowman's capsule

    c. Urine output

    d. Secretion of water in the nephron

20. Most diuretics act by blocking the reabsorption of _____ in the nephron.

    a. Large proteins

    b. Potassium

    c. Electrolytes

    d. Sodium

21. Which of the following is the most effective class of diuretics?

    a. Loop/high-ceiling

    b. Thiazides

    c. Osmotic

    d. Potassium-sparing

22. Blocking the reabsorption of sodium keeps more water in the filtrate. What effect does this have on urine flow?

    a. No effect

    b. Increased flow

    c. Decreased flow

    d. Increased or decreased flow, depending on lifestyle factors

23. When administering diuretics, the nurse should know that which of the following is a relatively common and serious side effect?

    a. Edema

    b. Hyperkalemia

    c. Dehydration

    d. Hypertension

24. Which of the following is an adverse effect specific to the *loop* class of diuretics?

    a. Hepatotoxicity

    b. Ototoxicity

    c. Dehydration

    d. Acidosis

25. The most widely prescribed class of diuretics is:

    a. Loop/high-ceiling

    b. Potassium-sparing

    c. Carbonic anhydrase inhibitors

    d. Thiazides

26. What is the primary indication for thiazide diuretics?

    a. Mild to moderate hypertension

    b. End-stage renal disease

    c. Dehydration

    d. Fluid loss

27. The nurse should teach patients that the intake of potassium-rich foods should NOT be increased during therapy with:

    a. Furosemide (Lasix)

    b. Chlorothiazide (Diuril)

    c. Spironolactone (Aldactone)

    d. Acetazolamide (Diamox)

28. Spironolactone acts by inhibiting:

    a. Aldosterone

    b. Carbonic anhydrase

    c. Potassium reabsorption in the distal tubule

    d. Sodium reabsorption in the loop of Henle

29. Which diuretic is prescribed specifically to decrease intraocular fluid pressure in patients with open-angle glaucoma?

    a. Torsemide (Demadex)

    b. Triamterene (Dyrenium)

    c. Chlorthalidone (Hygroton)

    d. Acetazolamide (Diamox)

30. Alkalosis begins to develop at a pH above:

    a. 6.5

    b. 7.0

    c. 7.35

    d. 7.45

31. When assessing for possible acidosis, the nurse should look for signs and symptoms related to which body system?

    a. Gastrointestinal (GI)

    b. CNS

    c. Renal

    d. Cardiovascular

32. Which drug can be administered by the nurse to reverse alkalosis?

    a. Sodium bicarbonate

    b. Sodium chloride combined with potassium chloride

    c. Lithium carbonate

    d. Aluminum hydroxide

33. Which of the following is a preferred drug for correcting acidosis?

    a. Sodium bicarbonate

    b. Sodium chloride

    c. Ammonium chloride

    d. Potassium chloride

34. Small inorganic molecules possessing a positive or negative charge are called:

    a. Acids

    b. Bases

    c. Electrolytes

    d. Colloids

35. Which of the following is a preferred drug for treating or preventing hypokalemia?

    a. Sodium bicarbonate

    b. Sodium chloride

    c. Ammonium chloride

    d. Potassium chloride

36. When administering oral potassium chloride, the health care provider should know that the most common adverse effect is:

    a. Drowsiness

    b. Nausea and vomiting

    c. Hypoglycemia

    d. Muscle weakness and fatigue

37. In severe cases, serum potassium levels may be quickly lowered by administration of:

    a. Glucose and insulin

    b. Furosemide (Lasix)

    c. Acetazolamide (Diamox)

    d. Sodium bicarbonate

38. Which of the following is a potential cause of acidosis?

    a. Kidney failure

    b. Ingestion of excess sodium bicarbonate

    c. Hyperventilation due to asthma, anxiety, or high altitude

    d. Diuretics that cause potassium depletion

39. Which of the following is a potential cause of alkalosis?

    a. Hypoventilation or shallow breathing

    b. Severe vomiting

    c. Severe diarrhea

    d. Diabetes mellitus

40. Hyponatremia is a deficiency of:

    a. Bicarbonate

    b. Sodium

    c. Magnesium

    d. Chloride

41. The nurse should teach patients that potassium supplements should be taken:

    a. With no other medications

    b. 1 hour before or 2 hours after a meal

    c. With a meal

    d. In the morning, on awakening

DO YOU REMEMBER?

42. Indapamide (Lozol) is a thiazide-like diuretic that is chemically related to sulfonamides. Sulfonamides are also used to treat:

    a. Peptic ulcers

    b. Viral infections

    c. Bacterial infections

    d. Anxiety

43. Scopolamine (Transderm-Scop) is an anticholinergic drug primarily used for:

    a. Dysrhythmias

    b. Hypertension

    c. Inflammation

    d. Motion sickness

44. A patient taking simvastatin is most likely being treated for:

    a. Hyperlipidemia

    b. Mild to moderate pain

    c. Myocardial infarction

    d. Insomnia

45. A patient is taking Hyzaar, a combination drug containing hydrochlorothiazide and losartan. This patient is likely being treated for:

    a. Shock

    b. Hypertension

    c. Parkinson's disease

    d. Migraines

46. Schedule V drugs are those that:

    a. Have a potential for abuse

    b. Are safe to take during pregnancy

    c. Have only minor side effects

    d. Are not yet approved by the Food and Drug Administration (FDA)

CASE STUDY APPLICATIONS

47. Mr. S is an active 56-year-old who was diagnosed with hypertension 12 months ago. At that time, he was placed on verapamil (Calan), hydrochlorothiazide (Microzide), and oral potassium chloride. He has not returned to your office since the initial diagnosis. During the past 12 months, he has reduced his weight from 280 lb to 198 lb using a rigorous exercise and diet program. Although he is proud of his lifestyle changes, he is complaining of fatigue, dizziness, heart palpitations, and muscle weakness.

    a. Give the rationale for each of the drugs initially prescribed for Mr. S.

    b. Can you offer a pharmacologic explanation for Mr. S's symptoms?

    c. What are some therapeutic options?

48. Ms. S, the wife of the patient in Question 47, also decided to lose weight, although she chose a plan that eliminated almost all dietary carbohydrates. She has been taking hydrochlorothiazide and aspirin for her arthritis and her husband's potassium chloride. After 2 weeks, she can no longer endure the stomach pain, nausea, and cramping. Her husband reports that his wife has shown considerable fatigue and sleepiness. Her stools have been black for the past week.

    a. Can you offer a pharmacologic explanation for Ms. S's symptoms?

    b. What are some therapeutic options?

CHAPTER 24

DRUGS FOR INFLAMMATION AND IMMUNE MODULATION

LEARNING OUTCOMES

To view the objectives, please refer to the textbook or MyNursingKit™ at www.mynursingkit.com.

TRUE/FALSE

For Questions 1–4, choose T for true or F for false.

T F 1. Biologic response modifiers are administered to boost natural immune responses.

T F 2. The primary class of drugs used to treat severe inflammation is the nonsteroidal anti-inflammatory drug (NSAID) class.

T F 3. Long-term therapy with glucocorticoids can result in Cushing's syndrome.

T F 4. Vaccines are effective at preventing a number of diseases, including HIV infection.

FILL IN THE BLANK

From the text, find the correct word(s) to complete the statement(s).

5. _____ occurs when preformed antibodies are transferred or "donated" from one person to another.

6. Immunosuppressants are effective at inhibiting a patient's immune system but must be monitored carefully because loss of immune function can lead to _____.

7. The central purpose of inflammation is to _____.

8. B cells and antibodies are associated with _____ immunity.

EXPLORE **PEARSON mynursing**

www.mynursingkit.com

MyNursingKit is your one stop for online chapter review materials and resources. Prepare for success with additional NCLEX®-style practice questions, interactive assignments and activities, web links, animations and videos, and more! Register your access code from the front of your book at www.mynursingkit.com.

9. When B cells encounter their specific antigen, they become _____ cells and secrete large quantities of _____.

10. Medications used to avoid tissue rejection following an organ transplant are called _____.

MATCHING

For Questions 11–20, match the drug in Column I with its primary class in Column II.

Column I	**Column II**
11. _____ Dexamethasone (Decadron)	a. NSAID
12. _____ Fenoprofen (Nalfon)	b. Systemic (oral) glucocorticoid
13. _____ Cyclosporine (Sandimmune, Neoral)	c. Immunosuppressant
14. _____ Oxaprozin (Daypro)	d. Biologic response modifier
15. _____ Levamisole (Ergamisole)	
16. _____ Tacrolimus (Prograf)	
17. _____ Prednisolone (Delta-Cortef)	
18. _____ Basiliximab (Simulect)	
19. _____ Celecoxib (Celebrex)	
20. _____ Muromonab-CD3 (Orthoclone OKT3)	

MULTIPLE CHOICE

21. The nurse should not administer hydrocortisone to a patient experiencing:

    a. An active infection associated with inflammation

    b. Pain associated with inflammation

    c. Nasal congestion

    d. Hypertension

22. Histamine is a potent:

    a. Vasodilator

    b. Vasoconstrictor

    c. Sympathomimetic

    d. Cardiotonic agent

23. Rapid release of histamine on a massive scale throughout the body is responsible for:

    a. Irreversible inhibition of cyclooxygenase

    b. Allergic rhinitis

    c. Immunosuppression

    d. Anaphylaxis

24. Foreign agents that elicit a specific immune response are called:

    a. Immunoglobulins

    b. Cytokines

    c. Antigens

    d. Antibodies

25. The primary function of plasma cells is to secrete:

    a. Complement

    b. Histamine

    c. Antibodies

    d. Cytokines

26. Memory B cells remember the initial antigen interaction and secrete high levels of antibodies in approximately:

    a. 2–3 hours

    b. 2–3 days

    c. 2–3 weeks

    d. 2–3 months

27. Which of the following drugs does NOT possess anti-inflammatory action?

    a. Aspirin

    b. Ibuprofen

    c. Acetaminophen

    d. COX-2 inhibitor

28. Aspirin acts by causing the irreversible inhibition of:

    a. Prostaglandin synthase

    b. Mast cells

    c. HMG-CoA reductase

    d. Cyclooxygenase

29. The nurse should teach patients that the most common adverse effects from high-dose aspirin therapy relate to which body system?

    a. Gastrointestinal (GI)

    b. Cardiovascular

    c. Endocrine

    d. Nervous

30. The primary advantage of the selective COX-2 inhibitors over aspirin is that they:

    a. Are less expensive

    b. Are more effective

    c. Have fewer adverse effects on the digestive system

    d. Have greater anticoagulant ability

31. Compared with aspirin, naproxen (Naprosyn) has _____ ability to relieve pain and reduce fever.

    a. Greater

    b. Less

    c. The same

    d. No

32. Which class of drugs has the potential to suppress the normal functions of the adrenal gland if given for long periods?

    a. NSAIDs

    b. Biologic response modifiers

    c. Immunosuppressants

    d. Glucocorticoids

33. Alternate-day therapy is common with which class of medications?

    a. Systemic glucocorticoids

    b. Biologic response modifiers

    c. Immunosuppressants

    d. Intranasal glucocorticoids

34. Which of the following drug classes is most effective at relieving severe inflammation?

    a. NSAIDs

    b. Systemic glucocorticoids

    c. Opioids

    d. COX-2 inhibitors

35. Which of the following drug classes would the nurse administer to avoid transplant rejection?

    a. COX-2 inhibitors

    b. Opioids

    c. Immunosuppressants

    d. Systemic glucocorticoids

36. Which of the following drugs produces its therapeutic effects by inhibiting T cells?

    a. Cyclosporine (Sandimmune)

    b. Prednisone

    c. Aspirin

    d. Celecoxib (Celebrex)

37. The health care provider should teach patients that the primary adverse effects from cyclosporine occur in the:

    a. Immune system

    b. Lung

    c. GI tract

    d. Kidney

38. Which of the following is NOT a type of vaccine suspension?

    a. Live microbes

    b. Killed microbes

    c. Microbes that are alive but attenuated

    d. Bacterial toxins

39. The nurse should teach patients that the purpose of a vaccine is to:

    a. Treat active infections

    b. Prevent inflammation should an infection occur

    c. Prevent infections from occurring

    d. Suppress the immune system so that hypersensitivity to antigens does not occur

40. A toxoid is best classified as a(n):

    a. Vaccine

    b. Immunosuppressant

    c. Anti-inflammatory agent

    d. Antigen

DO YOU REMEMBER?

41. Hydrochlorothiazide is one of the most frequently prescribed:

    a. Diuretics

    b. Antiseizure drugs

    c. Antidysrhythmics

    d. Electrolytes

42. More frequent and potentially severe adverse effects will be observed when a drug is given by which route?

    a. Oral

    b. IM

    c. IV

    d. SC

43. What is the most common indication for phenytoin (Dilantin)?

    a. Bipolar disorder

    b. Schizophrenia

    c. Migraines

    d. Seizures

44. Which organ is responsible for the "first-pass" effect?

    a. Liver

    b. Kidneys

    c. Brain

    d. Small intestine

45. Which of the following drugs is classified as an opioid?

    a. Hydralazine (Apresoline)

    b. Hydrocodone (Hycodan)

    c. Hydrocortisone

    d. Hydrochlorothiazide (Macrozide)

CASE STUDY APPLICATIONS

46. Mr. E is an 18-year-old patient who arrives at the physician's office with a toothache. The nurse observes an abscess surrounding a molar that is red, swollen, and inflamed. Because of the patient's fever, the nurse suspects that a bacterial infection from the abscess has spread throughout the body. The following medications are prescribed.

    Ampicillin
    Empirin with Codeine #2
    Ketoprofen (Orudis)

    a. What is the therapeutic rationale for the medications prescribed by the physician?

    b. Why did the physician not prescribe a glucocorticoid to reduce the inflammation?

47. Certain cells in the immune system can interact with antigens and produce inflammation. The inflammatory process itself, however, can occur without the direction of the immune system.

    a. How does the inflammatory response differ from the immune response?

    b. Are the drugs used to treat an abnormally strong inflammatory response also used to treat hyperresponses of the immune system?

CHAPTER 25

DRUGS FOR BACTERIAL INFECTIONS

LEARNING OUTCOMES

To view the objectives, please refer to the textbook or
MyNursingKit™ at www.mynursingkit.com.

TRUE/FALSE

For Questions 1–9, choose T for true or F for false.

T F 1. Bacteria that appear a distinctive purple color after applying a violet stain are called gram negative.

T F 2. Bacteriocidal drugs kill infectious organisms, whereas bacteriostatic drugs slow down their growth.

T F 3. Acquired resistance develops from taking too high a dose of antibiotics and is less likely when smaller doses are administered over a longer period.

T F 4. Large numbers of resistant bacterial strains limit the therapeutic usefulness of many penicillins.

T F 5. Cephalosporins have a different mechanism of action than the penicillins.

T F 6. Patients may experience photosensitivity when taking tetracyclines.

T F 7. Macrolides are an effective antibiotic class; however, patients must take these drugs for a longer time due to their relatively short half-life.

T F 8. Ototoxicity is a common adverse effect of erythromycin and clarithromycin (Biaxin).

T F 9. Fluoroquinolones are effective against *Pseudomonas*, a microorganism often responsible for urinary tract and skin infections.

 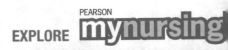

FILL IN THE BLANK

From the text, find the correct word(s) to complete the statement(s).

10. A highly _____ microbe is one that can produce disease when present in minute numbers.

11. Genetic errors called _____ commonly occur in bacterial cells and result in drug resistance.

12. A(n) _____ infection is one acquired in a hospital setting.

13. A(n) _____ is a type of infection that occurs secondarily to anti-infective therapy.

14. _____ is an enzyme secreted by bacteria, which limits the therapeutic usefulness of penicillins.

15. One of the most widely prescribed classes of antibiotics, similar in structure and function to the penicillins, is _____.

16. Augmentin, Timentin, and Unasyn are combination drugs that contain a penicillin and a _____.

17. Narrow-spectrum antibiotics, called _____, are useful for the treatment of serious gram-negative infections, but they have the potential for producing ear and kidney toxicity.

MATCHING

For Questions 18–28, match the drug in Column I with its pharmacologic category in Column II.

Column I

18. _____ Amoxicillin (Amoxil, Trimox)

19. _____ Ciprofloxacin (Cipro)

20. _____ Cefepime (Maxipime)

21. _____ Gentamycin (Garamycin)

22. _____ Neomycin

23. _____ Erythromycin (E-mycin, Erythrocin)

24. _____ Doxycycline (Vibramycin)

25. _____ Cephalexin (Keflex)

26. _____ Ampicillin (Principen)

27. _____ Rifampin (Rifadin, Rimactane)

28. _____ Vancomycin (Vancocin)

Column II

a. Penicillin

b. Cephalosporin

c. Tetracycline

d. Macrolide

e. Aminoglycoside

f. Fluoroquinolone or miscellaneous

g. Antitubercular agent

For Questions 29–36, match the organism in Column I with its disease(s) in Column II.

Column I

29. _____ *Vibrio*

30. _____ *Streptococci*

31. _____ *Pneumococci*

32. _____ *Rickettsia*

33. _____ *Klebsiella*

34. _____ *Borrelia*

35. _____ *Escherichia*

36. _____ *Chlamydia*

Column II

a. Venereal disease, endometriosis

b. Cholera

c. Traveler's diarrhea, urinary tract infection (UTI), endometriosis

d. Pharyngitis, pneumonia, skin infections, septicemia, endocarditis

e. Lyme disease

f. Rocky mountain spotted fever

g. Pneumonia, otitis media, meningitis, bacteremia, endocarditis

h. Pneumonia, UTI

MULTIPLE CHOICE

37. An antibiotic with a broad spectrum is one that:

    a. Produces a large number of side effects

    b. Is effective against a small number of organisms

    c. Is effective against a large number of organisms

    d. Has a high potency

38. Bacteriocidal drugs are those that:

    a. Have a high potency

    b. Have high effectiveness

    c. Kill the infectious agent

    d. Slow the growth of the infectious agent

39. What advantage does amoxicillin (Amoxil, Trimox) have over penicillin G?

    a. It is less expensive.

    b. It has greater absorption.

    c. It has fewer side effects.

    d. It has penicillinase resistance.

40. Which antibiotic class is usually reserved for serious UTIs because of the potential for ototoxicity and nephrotoxicity?

    a. Erythromycins

    b. Aminoglycosides

    c. Tetracyclines

    d. Sulfonamides

41. Which antibiotic is known as the "last chance" drug for those with resistant infections?

    a. Clarithromycin (Biaxin)

    b. Dicloxacillin

    c. Vancomycin (Vancocin)

    d. Trimethoprim-sulfamethoxazole (Bactrim, Septra)

42. Which of the following would most likely be used for a patient allergic to penicillin?

    a. Clindamycin (Cleocin)

    b. Amoxicillin (Amoxil)

    c. Sulfisoxazole (Gantrisin)

    d. Erythromycin (E-mycin)

43. A drug that is effective against a large number of different species of bacteria is said to:

    a. Be bacteriocidal

    b. Be bacteriostatic

    c. Have a wide spectrum of activity

    d. Have a narrow spectrum of activity

44. The nurse should teach patients that photosensitivity and teeth discoloration are potential adverse effects of:

    a. Aminoglycosides

    b. Metronidazole (Flagyl)

    c. Cephalosporins

    d. Tetracyclines

45. A drug of choice for the treatment of *M. tuberculosis* is:

    a. Erythromycin (E-mycin, Erythrocin)

    b. Gentamicin (Garamycin)

    c. Vancomycin (Vancocin)

    d. Isoniazid (INH)

46. An antibiotic responsible for causing "red-man syndrome" as an adverse effect is:

    a. Cefotaxime (Claforan)

    b. Tetracycline HCI (Sumycin, others)

    c. Erythromycin (E-mycin, Erythrocin)

    d. Vancomycin (Vancocin)

47. Drug therapy of tuberculosis differs from that of most other infections because:

    a. Patients with tuberculosis have no symptoms.

    b. Mycobacteria have a cell wall that is resistant to penetration by anti-infective drugs.

    c. Patients usually require therapy for a shorter period.

    d. Antituberculosis drugs are used extensively for treating active disease, not preventing it.

48. The purpose of culture and sensitivity testing is to:

    a. Prevent an infection, a practice called chemoprophylaxis

    b. Determine which antibiotic is most effective against the infecting microorganism

    c. Identify bacteria that have acquired resistance

    d. Promote the development of drug-resistant bacterial strains by killing the bacteria sensitive to a drug

49. Which of the following types of antibiotics are more likely to cause superinfections?

    a. Narrow-spectrum antibiotics

    b. Broad-spectrum antibiotics

    c. The original penicillin

    d. Bacteriostatic drugs

50. Which antibiotic class is one of the oldest, safest, and effective although widespread resistance has developed to the drugs?

    a. Penicillins

    b. Tetracyclines

    c. Macrolides

    d. Aminoglycosides

51. Factors contributing to acquired resistance include:

    a. Errors during replication of bacterial DNA

    b. Overuse of antibiotics

    c. Not taking antibiotic therapy for the prescribed length of time

    d. a and b

DO YOU REMEMBER?

52. Which local anesthetic drug might interfere with the antibacterial activity of some sulfonamide drugs?

    a. Benzocaine (Americaine)

    b. Tetracaine (Pontocaine)

    c. Bupivacaine (Marcaine)

    d. Lidocaine (Xylocaine)

53. Which of the following actions might influence antibiotic absorption within the stomach?

    a. Taking an antacid along with the antibiotic

    b. Drinking a glass of water with the antibiotic

    c. Taking an antibiotic suspension without shaking up the medicine vial

    d. Taking the antibiotic just before going to bed

54. If convulsive seizures were to develop with antibiotic therapy, which of the following symptoms would most likely NOT be observed?

    a. Jerking muscular movements

    b. Difficulty breathing and biting the tongue

    c. A blank stare with psychotic symptoms

    d. Loss of bladder control

55. Following oral administration, chlorpromazine (Thorazine) is rapidly inactivated by the liver. This inactivation is referred to as:

    a. Enterohepatic recirculation

    b. First-pass effect

    c. Gastric-hepatic barrier

    d. Enzyme induction

56. Which of the following terms is NOT associated with the drug levodopa (Dopar)?

    a. Anticholinergic

    b. Anti-Parkinson's disease agent

    c. Dopamine

    d. Sympathomimetic

CASE STUDY APPLICATIONS

57. For several years, Ms. P has been taking antibiotics off and on for kidney infections. She has been warned that, the more antibiotics she takes, the more likely it is that she will develop an infection that is resistant to that drug. Explain why Ms. P should be careful, and point out special precautions she should take because of her persistent problem.

58. Mr. N has been diagnosed with bacterial pneumonia and has been treated with a broad-spectrum antibiotic until it can be determined exactly what has caused the ailment. What actions should be considered in trying to provide more specific drug therapy for this patient?

CHAPTER 26

DRUGS FOR FUNGAL, VIRAL, AND PARASITIC DISEASES

LEARNING OUTCOMES

To view the objectives, please refer to the textbook or MyNursingKit™ at www.mynursingkit.com.

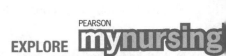
TRUE/FALSE

For Questions 1–7, choose T for true or F for false.

T   F   1. Systemic mycoses are fungal infections affecting the skin, nails, and mucous membranes, such as the oral cavity.

T   F   2. Ketoconazole (Nizoral) has become a preferred drug for less severe mycoses and for the prophylaxis of fungal infections.

T   F   3. The major adverse effects of superficial antifungal medications are minor skin irritation or, when given orally, diarrhea, nausea, and vomiting.

T   F   4. Antiviral drugs are not usually specific to one virus; rather, they are effective against many different kinds of viral infections.

T   F   5. Highly active antiretroviral therapy (HAART) is the main form of treatment for disorders caused by herpes simplex viruses.

T   F   6. Acyclovir (Zovirax) acts by inhibiting viral deoxyribonucleic acid (DNA) synthesis.

T   F   7. *Entamoeba histolytica*, the organism responsible for malaria, is best treated with metronidazole (Flagyl).

FILL IN THE BLANK

From the text, find the correct word(s) to complete the statement(s).

8. The basic structure of a virus includes its outer protein coat, called the _____, and its inner genetic material in the form of _____ or _____.

9. _____ is a class of medications used to block components of the replication cycle of the HIV.

10. A(n) _____ is a virus that causes uncomfortable symptoms associated with the common cold.

11. The first antiviral medication used to treat AIDS was _____.

12. Osteltamivir (Tamiflu) and zanamivir (Relenza) are examples of a newer class of drugs, called the _____, used to treat active influenza infections.

13. The antiviral drug that has been available to prevent and treat influenza for many years is _____.

14. The preferred drug for the treatment of the herpesvirus infections is _____.

15. The drug of choice for most forms of amebiasis is _____.

MATCHING

For Questions 16–21, match the name of the fungus in Column I with whether it usually causes a systemic or topical infection in Column II.

Column I	Column II
16. _____ *Aspergillus fumigatus*	a. Systemic infection
17. _____ *Epidermophyton floccosum*	b. Topical infection
18. _____ *Coccidioides immitis*	
19. _____ *Histoplasma capsulatum*	
20. _____ *Sporothrix schenckii*	
21. _____ *Mucorales*	

For Questions 22–27, match the antifungal drug in Column I with its indication in Column II.

Column I	Column II
22. _____ Butoconazole (Femstat)	a. Skin mycoses
23. _____ Econazole (Spectazole)	b. Ringworm, skin, and nail infections
24. _____ Flucytosine (Ancobon)	c. Vaginal mycoses
25. _____ Griseofulvin (Fulvicin)	d. Severe systemic infections
26. _____ Nystatin (Mycostatin, others)	e. Candidiasis
27. _____ Undeclyenic acid (Fungi-Nail, Gordochom, others)	f. Athlete's foot, diaper rash

MULTIPLE CHOICE

28. Systemic mycoses often require which of the following treatments?

    a. Topical agents only

    b. Oral medications only

    c. Parenteral medications only

    d. Oral and parenteral medications

29. Treatment of which of the following disorders does NOT usually include systemic antifungal drugs?

    a. Extensive burns

    b. Cancer

    c. Organ transplant

    d. Influenza

30. Oral drugs administered for systemic fungal infections include all of the following EXCEPT:

    a. Fluconazole (Diflucan)

    b. Itraconazole (Sporonox)

    c. Ketoconazole (Nizoral)

    d. Amphotericin B (Fungizone, others)

31. Which of the following medications used to treat candidiasis is available in a wide variety of formulations, including cream, ointment, powder, tablets, and lozenges?

    a. Butenafine (Mentax)

    b. Ciclopiroxolamine (Loprox)

    c. Nystatin (Mycostatin)

    d. Haloprogin (Halotex)

32. The nurse should teach patients that one of the most common side effects of systemic amphotericin B (Fungizone, others) therapy is:

    a. Phlebitis

    b. Neurotoxicity

    c. Gastric reflux

    d. Dryness of the mouth

33. Superficial antifungal drugs are effective in all of the following cases EXCEPT:

    a. Nail infection

    b. Infections of the mucous membranes

    c. Suppressed immune system

    d. Infection of the scalp and hair

34. Which of the following drugs used to treat HIV/AIDS is a nonnucleoside reverse transcriptase inhibitor?

    a. Zidovudine (Retrovir, AZT)

    b. Nevirapine (Viramune)

    c. Lamivudine (Epivir, 3TC)

    d. Indinavir (Crixivan)

35. Acyclovir (Zovirax) is an effective treatment for all of the following viruses EXCEPT:

    a. Herpes simplex viruses (HSV) types 1 and 2

    b. Cytomegalovirus (CMV)

    c. Varicella-zoster virus

    d. Epstein-Barr virus

36. The best approach to influenza treatment is:

    a. Prevention through annual vaccinations

    b. Amantadine (Symmetrel)

    c. Oseltamivir (Tamiflu)

    d. Zanamivir (Relenza)

37. The purpose and expected outcome of HIV pharmacotherapy includes which of the following?

    a. Patients with HIV are able to live symptom-free much longer.

    b. The Food and Drug Administration (FDA) has approved over 16 new antiviral drugs for the cure of HIV.

    c. Drugs have been developed that treat only slowly mutating and less resistant HIV strains.

    d. Drugs have become available that treat the mother infected with HIV without much success to the newborn.

38. The goal of HAART is to:

    a. Increase the patient's quality of life

    b. Increase the patient's life span

    c. Reduce the plasma level of HIV to its lowest possible value

    d. All of the above

39. All of the following are drug classes used to treat HIV-AIDS EXCEPT:

    a. Nonnucleoside reverse transcriptase inhibitors (NNRTIs)

    b. Nucleoside reverse transcriptase inhibitors (NRTIs)

    c. Fusion inhibitors

    d. DNA synthesis inhibitors

40. One of the major toxic effects of zidovudine (Retrovir, AZT) is:

    a. Reduced numbers of red and white blood cells

    b. Painful inflammation of blood vessels at the site of infusion

    c. Nephrotoxicity

    d. b and c

41. The nurse would administer which of the following drugs for traveler's diarrhea?

    a. Doxycycline hyclate (Vibramycin)

    b. Mebendazole (Vermox)

    c. Chloroquine (Aralen)

    d. Metronidazole (Flagyl)

42. Which of the following medications was once commonly used for treating malaria but has been replaced by other antimalarials?

    a. Praziquantel (Biltricide)

    b. Quinine sulfate (Quinamm)

    c. Melarsoprol (Arsobal)

    d. Trimetrexate (Neutrexin)

43. Which of the following is the standard therapy for treating helminthes infections by *Ascaris*?

    a. Chloroquine (Aralen)

    b. Metronidazole (Flagyl)

    c. Mebendazole (Vermox)

    d. Rimantadine (Flumadine)

DO YOU REMEMBER?

44. When bacteria mutate and become resistant to antibiotics, what part of their physical makeup is altered?

    a. DNA

    b. Protein

    c. Beta-lactam ring

    d. Enzymes

45. Which of the following drugs or class of drugs induces hepatic microsomal enzymes, decreasing the effectiveness of some antiparasitic medication?

    a. Opioids

    b. Phenobarbital

    c. Aspirin

    d. Phenothiazines

46. Any drug that increases the renal reabsorption of an antiviral drug would:

    a. Increase the half-life of the medication

    b. Decrease the half-life of the medication

    c. Have no effect on the half-life of the medication

    d. Also increase excretion

47. A patient who is allergic to penicillin G may also be allergic to:

    a. Ampicillin

    b. Tetracycline

    c. Ciprofloxacin (Cipro)

    d. Vancomycin (Vancocin)

48. Ibuprofen is best classified as a(n):

   a. Salicylate

   b. Opioid

   c. Selective COX-2 inhibitor

   d. Nonsteroidal anti-inflammatory drug (NSAID)

CASE STUDY APPLICATIONS

49. Ms. B is pregnant and thinks she has vaginal candidiasis. The apparent infection is not serious, but it is a concern. What approach should Ms. B take to have this infection treated, and what precautions should be considered?

50. Mr. R is HIV positive and was told that combination drug therapy would be more effective for this disorder than a single drug. Why is this true?

CHAPTER 27

DRUGS FOR NEOPLASIA

LEARNING OUTCOMES

To view the objectives, please refer to the textbook or MyNursingKit™ at www.mynursingkit.com.

TRUE/FALSE

For Questions 1–9, choose T for true or F for false.

T   F   1. Malignant tumors are those that do not metastasize and rarely require drug treatment.

T   F   2. Medications from different chemotherapeutic classes are rarely combined when patients receive surgery or radiation treatment.

T   F   3. Resistance to antineoplastic drugs is not a phenomenon observed with cancer cells.

T   F   4. Specific dosing schedules have been found to increase the effectiveness of antineoplastic agents.

T   F   5. Alkylating agents interfere with aspects of the nucleic acid *metabolism* of rapidly growing tumor cells.

T   F   6. Some antibiotics have the ability to kill cancer cells.

T   F   7. Plant extracts are used for chemotherapy because they have relatively few adverse effects.

T   F   8. Corticosteroids, estrogens, and androgens are commonly used in cancer chemotherapy.

T   F   9. Biologic response modifiers differ from other chemotherapeutic agents in that they stimulate the patient's own immune system to fight the cancer cells.

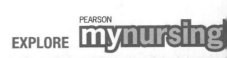

FILL IN THE BLANK

From the text, find the correct word(s) to complete the statement(s).

10. Drug therapy of cancer is sometimes called _____.

11. A number of treatment strategies have been found to increase the effectiveness of anticancer drugs, including _____, _____, _____, and _____.

12. A novel delivery method in which drugs are enclosed in small sacs, or vesicles, of lipids is called _____.

13. Bone marrow suppression is the most important adverse effect of a class of antineoplastic drugs called _____.

14. By blocking the synthesis of folic acid, a medication called _____ is able to inhibit replication in rapidly dividing cancer cells.

15. All antitumor antibiotics must be administered by the _____ route or through direct installation into a body cavity using a catheter.

16. Plant extracts that have been isolated to kill cancer cells include the _____, _____, and _____.

17. _____ help to limit the severe immunosuppressive effects of other anticancer drugs by stimulating the body's immune system.

MATCHING

For Questions 18–27, match the medication in Column I with its pharmacologic classification in Column II.

Column I	Column II
18. _____ Cyclophosphamide (Cytoxan)	a. Alkylating agent
19. _____ Fluorouracil (5-FU, Adrucil)	b. Antimetabolite
20. _____ Vincristine sulfate (Oncovin)	c. Antitumor antibiotic
21. _____ Methotrexate (Rheumatrex, Trexall)	d. Hormones and hormone antagonist
22. _____ Bleomycin (Blenoxane)	e. Plant extract
23. _____ Medroxyprogesterone (Provera)	f. Biologic response modifier or miscellaneous
24. _____ Etoposide (VePesid)	
25. _____ Tamoxifen (Nolvadex)	
26. _____ Levamisole (Ergamisol)	
27. _____ Streptozocin (Zanosar)	

MULTIPLE CHOICE

28. Antimetabolites act by:

    a. Changing the structure of deoxyribonucleic acid (DNA) in cancer cells

    b. Disrupting critical cell pathways in cancer cells

    c. Preventing cell division

    d. Activating the body's immune system

29. Bruising is a common side effect of chemotherapy, caused by a deficiency of:

    a. Platelets

    b. Red blood cells

    c. White blood cells

    d. Normal bacterial flora

30. The health care provider should teach patients that the probability of acquiring cancer may be reduced by adopting which of the following lifestyle changes?

    a. Examining the skin for abnormal lesions or changes to moles

    b. Exercising regularly and keeping body weight within normal guidelines

    c. Examining the body monthly for abnormal lumps

    d. All of the above

31. Which of the following statements regarding tumors is INCORRECT?

    a. Carcinomas are the most common type of neoplasm.

    b. Benign tumors are slow growing, do not metastasize, and rarely require drug treatment.

    c. Malignant tumors grow rapidly worse, become resistant to treatment, and normally result in death.

    d. The term *neoplasm* is often used interchangeably with *carcinogen*.

32. Which of the following is NOT a treatment approach to remove cancer?

    a. Surgery

    b. Radiation therapy

    c. Diet

    d. Drug therapy

33. Which of the following approaches would eliminate the maximum number of cancer cells with the least toxicity?

    a. Using multiple drugs in lower doses from different antineoplastic classes

    b. Increasing the concentration of different antineoplastic drugs from the same class

    c. Increasing the dose of one antineoplastic drug

    d. Combining radiation therapy with chemotherapy treatment

34. Which of the following would the nurse NOT expect to observe during chemotherapy with antineoplastic drugs?

    a. Alopecia

    b. Nausea

    c. Hypercholesterolemia

    d. Leukopenia

35. Which of the following acts by changing the shape of DNA and preventing it from functioning normally?

    a. Cyclophosphamide (Cytoxan)

    b. Methotrexate (Rheumatrex, Trexall)

    c. Doxorubicin (Adriamycin)

    d. Vincristine (Oncovin)

36. The primary drug therapy for AIDS-related Kaposi's sarcoma is:

    a. Mechlorethamine (Mustargen)

    b. Floxuridine (FUDR)

    c. Doxorubicin (Adriamycin)

    d. Teniposide (Vumon)

37. A chemotherapeutic agent extracted from the Pacific yew plant is:

    a. Mercaptopurine (6-MP, Purinethol)

    b. Paclitaxel (Taxol)

    c. Vinblastine sulfate (Velban)

    d. Flutamide (Eulexin)

38. The most serious limiting adverse effect of vincristine (Oncovin) is:

    a. Flulike symptoms

    b. Hepatotoxicity

    c. Neurotoxicity

    d. Immunosuppression

39. The preferred drug for treating breast cancer is:

    a. Carboplatin (Paraplatin)

    b. Pentostatin (Nipent)

    c. Epirubicin (Ellence)

    d. Tamoxifen citrate (Nolvadex)

40. Which anticancer drug is similar to the insecticide DDT?

    a. Interferon alfa 2 (Roferon-A, Intron A)

    b. Mitotane (Lysodren)

    c. Paclitaxel (Taxol)

    d. Irinotecan (Camptosar)

41. Which of the following drugs would the nurse administer for palliation of advanced cancer?

    a. Epirubicin (Ellence)

    b. Dacarbazine (DTIC-Dome)

    c. Ethinyl estradiol (Estinyl)

    d. Chlorambucil (Leukeran)

42. Which of the following drugs would NOT be used for treatment of prostate cancer?

    a. Vinorelbine (Navelbine)

    b. Megestrol (Megace)

    c. Bicalutamide (Casodex)

    d. Leuprolide (Lupron)

43. Which of the following drugs would the nurse administer for palliative treatment of malignant melanoma?

    a. Teniposide (Vumon)

    b. Idarubicin (Idamycin)

    c. Dactinomycin (Actinomycin D, Cosmegan)

    d. Hydroxyurea (Hydrea)

44. In a patient with cancer, the nurse would administer oprelvekin (Neumega) in order to:

    a. Kill the maximum number of cancer cells

    b. Protect normal cells from being killed by other chemotherapy agents

    c. Stimulate red blood cell production

    d. Stimulate platelet production

DO YOU REMEMBER?

45. Which of the following drugs would most likely displace an antineoplastic drug from protein binding sites in the plasma, thus increasing its effect?

    a. Nonsteroidal anti-inflammatory drugs (NSAIDs)

    b. Sedative-hypnotics

    c. Antidepressants

    d. Calcium channel blockers

46. Heart failure is sometimes observed with antineoplastic drugs. The nurse should assess for which of the following symptoms in this patient?

    a. Hypokalemia

    b. Peripheral edema

    c. Dehydration

    d. Dysrhythmias

47. Glycoprotein IIb/IIIa inhibitors are used to treat:

    a. Blood coagulation disorders

    b. Depression

    c. Tuberculosis

    d. HIV/AIDS

48. Divalproex (Depakote) is useful in the pharmacotherapy of migraines, bipolar disorder, and:

    a. Schizophrenia

    b. Angina

    c. Dysrhythmias

    d. Seizures

49. Indomethacin (Indocin) is a medication that prevents prostaglandin synthesis. It would most likely be used to treat:

    a. Fungal infections

    b. Pain and inflammation

    c. Hypotension

    d. Alzheimer's disease

CASE STUDY APPLICATIONS

50. Mr. U is receiving chemotherapy for prostate cancer and has been told that chemotherapy drugs are expected to kill 99% of tumor cells. However, remaining cells could cause his tumor to return and produce significant damage. Explain how this might be prevented.

51. Ms. H has been receiving chemotherapy for 3 weeks and has experienced a number of side effects, including nausea, vomiting, infections, and anorexia. Explain how the nurse could help minimize these effects.

CHAPTER 28

DRUGS FOR RESPIRATORY DISORDERS

LEARNING OUTCOMES

To view the objectives, please refer to the textbook or MyNursingKit™ at www.mynursingkit.com.

TRUE/FALSE

For Questions 1–5, choose T for true or F for false.

T   F   1. The primary use of glucocorticoids, such as beclomethasone (Beconase AQ), in asthma is to *terminate* acute asthmatic attacks.

T   F   2. H_1-receptor blockers are commonly called antihistamines.

T   F   3. Compared with their oral counterparts, *inhaled* beta-adrenergic agents produce less toxicity because only small amounts of the drugs are absorbed.

T   F   4. Systemic side effects are rare when using intranasal glucocorticoids.

T   F   5. When administered intranasally, sympathomimetics do not produce rebound congestion.

FILL IN THE BLANK

From the text, find the correct word(s) to complete the statement(s).

6. Small machines that vaporize a liquid drug into a fine mist that can be inhaled are called _____.

7. Drug classes used to prevent allergic rhinitis include _____, _____, and _____.

8. Because the sympathomimetics relieve only nasal congestion, they are often combined with _____ in order to control the sneezing and tearing of allergic rhinitis.

9. Oral and intranasal _____ are effective at relieving nasal congestion due to the common cold.

MULTIPLE CHOICE

10. Which of the following is NOT characteristic of asthma?

    a. Inflammation

    b. Infection

    c. Bronchoconstriction

    d. Dyspnea

11. Which of the following classes would LEAST likely be prescribed for asthma?

    a. Beta$_2$-agents

    b. Xanthines

    c. Glucocorticoids

    d. Beta blockers

12. Which of the following classes are the MOST effective drugs for relieving acute bronchospasm?

    a. Beta$_2$-adrenergic agents

    b. Mast cell stabilizers

    c. Xanthines

    d. Anticholinergics

13. The nurse would NOT administer salmeterol (Serevent) to terminate an acute bronchospasm because the drug:

    a. Is not absorbed orally

    b. Takes too long to act

    c. Affects only beta$_1$-receptors

    d. Causes too much central nervous system (CNS) stimulation

14. For the prophylaxis of nonpersistent asthma, glucocorticoids are most commonly administered by which route?

    a. Oral

    b. Topical

    c. Intranasal

    d. Intradermal

15. Glucocorticoids improve asthma symptoms by:

    a. Causing bronchodilation

    b. Suppressing inflammation

    c. Blocking histamine release

    d. Drying bronchial secretions

16. During long-term treatment with oral glucocorticoids, the nurse should assess for which serious adverse effect?

    a. Rebound congestion

    b. Hypertension

    c. Cancer

    d. Adrenal atrophy/insufficiency

17. The nurse should assess for candidiasis of the throat during therapy with which class of medications?

    a. Inhaled glucocorticoids

    b. Mast cell stabilizers

    c. Beta$_2$-agents

    d. Mucolytics

18. The primary use of mast cell inhibitors in the treatment of asthma is to:

    a. Terminate acute asthmatic attacks

    b. Prevent asthmatic attacks

    c. Reduce secretions

    d. Reduce infections

19. The primary action of an antitussive is to:

    a. Suppress the cough reflex

    b. Dry bronchial secretions

    c. Block histamine release

    d. Reduce the viscosity of bronchial secretions

20. The primary action of an expectorant is to:

    a. Suppress the cough reflex

    b. Dry bronchial secretions

    c. Reduce inflammation

    d. Reduce the viscosity of bronchial secretions

21. The most effective antitussives are from which drug class?

    a. Opioids

    b. Glucocorticoids

    c. Beta$_2$-agents

    d. Nonsteroidal anti-inflammatory drugs (NSAIDs)

22. For the treatment of allergies, the newer antihistamines are an improvement over the older, more traditional antihistamines because they:

    a. Are less sedating

    b. Are more effective

    c. Are more potent

    d. Cause less gastrointestinal (GI) irritation

23. Symptoms of motion sickness are often treated with:

    a. H_1-receptor blockers

    b. H_2-receptor blockers

    c. Immunosuppressants

    d. Intranasal glucocorticoids

24. Which of the following drugs is often combined with analgesics and decongestants in over-the-counter (OTC) cold medications?

    a. Fluticasone (Flonase)

    b. Fexofenadine (Allegra)

    c. Diphenhydramine (Benadryl)

    d. Prednisone (Meticorten)

25. Which of the following is NOT an indication for diphenhydramine?

    a. Parkinson's disease

    b. Peptic ulcer

    c. Motion sickness

    d. Insomnia

26. Glucocorticoids have joined antihistamines as preferred drugs in the treatment of allergic rhinitis. For this disorder, glucocorticoids are administered via which route?

    a. Oral

    b. Topical

    c. IM

    d. Intranasal

27. The nurse should teach patients that the most frequently reported side effect of intranasal glucocorticoids is:

    a. Sinus congestion

    b. Tachycardia

    c. Burning sensation in the nose

    d. Dry mouth

28. Which of the following autonomic classes are commonly used to dry the nasal mucosa for patients with colds and allergies?

    a. Sympathomimetics

    b. Anticholinergics

    c. Cholinergics

    d. Beta-adrenergic blockers

29. Intranasal drugs, such as oxymetazoline (Afrin), produce an effective response in:

    a. Less than 5 minutes

    b. 20 minutes

    c. 1 to 2 hours

    d. 2 to 3 days

30. Rebound congestion is most common with which class of medications?

    a. Antihistamines

    b. Intranasal sympathomimetics

    c. Intranasal glucocorticoids

    d. NSAIDs

DO YOU REMEMBER?

31. The nurse would not administer selective beta$_1$-agents for asthma because:

    a. There are no beta$_1$-receptors in bronchial smooth muscle.

    b. They cannot be delivered by the inhalation route.

    c. They cause bronchoconstriction.

    d. Their duration of action is too short.

32. Trizivir is a combination drug that contains abacavir, lamivudine, and zidovudine. This medication is most likely used to treat:

    a. Bacterial infections

    b. Fungal infections

    c. Herpes infections

    d. HIV/AIDS

33. Which of the following is a drug of choice for opioid overdose?

    a. Methadone (Dolophine)

    b. Epinephrine (Adrenalin)

    c. Naloxone (Narcan)

    d. Dobutamine (Dobutrex)

34. Which of the following drugs has analgesic, anti-inflammatory, and antipyretic activity?

    a. Morphine sulfate

    b. Aspirin

    c. Acetaminophen

    d. Vicodin (hydrocodone with acetaminophen)

35. The use of penicillin G has declined over the past decade, primarily because:

    a. There are less expensive alternatives.

    b. More people are becoming allergic to the drug.

    c. Other antibiotics are available that cause fewer side effects.

    d. Widespread microbial resistance has developed.

CASE STUDY APPLICATIONS

36. Mr. H arrives in the emergency department (ED) extremely short of breath and quite anxious. He has a history of asthma and hypertension. His blood pressure is elevated. Mr. H claims that the beclomethasone (Beconase) inhaler that he was given 2 months ago has been unable to ease his shortness of breath. The physician prescribes lorazepam (Ativan) and metaproterenol (Alupent) while Mr. H is in the ED. Prior to his hospital visit, Mr. H had been taking the following medications:

    Beclomethasone (Beconase) inhaler
    Propranolol (Inderal)

    a. Give the therapeutic rationales for the two drugs taken by Mr. H *prior* to the ED visit.

    b. Explain how beclomethasone and propranolol may have contributed to Mr. H's symptoms.

    c. Give the therapeutic rationales for the two drugs taken by Mr. H *during* his ED visit.

37. Ms. A is concerned because her 8-year-old daughter, Michelle, is experiencing severe flu symptoms. She is complaining of a fever of 101.2, fatigue, and severe nasal congestion. Today she started a cough, producing small amounts of thick sputum. Ms. A calls the physician, who prescribes the following medications:

    Novahistine expectorant
    Acetaminophen

    a. Name the ingredients in Novahistine and explain the function of each.

    b. What is the therapeutic rationale for acetaminophen? Why was acetaminophen prescribed instead of aspirin?

CHAPTER 29

DRUGS FOR GASTROINTESTINAL DISORDERS

LEARNING OUTCOMES

To view the objectives, please refer to the textbook or
MyNursingKit™ at www.mynursingkit.com.

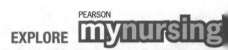

TRUE/FALSE

For Questions 1–5, choose T for true or F for false.

T F 1. Laxatives generally produce a more natural and gentle
       bowel movement than cathartics.

T F 2. Gastric ulcers are less common than duodenal ulcers.

T F 3. Anorexia, weight loss, and vomiting are more common
       with gastric ulcers than with duodenal ulcers.

T F 4. All H_2-receptor blockers are antihistamines, but not all antihistamines are H_2-receptor blockers.

T F 5. Cimetidine (Tagamet) and famotidine (Pepcid) act by neutralizing acid to raise the pH of the stomach.

FILL IN THE BLANK

From the text, find the correct word(s) to complete the statement(s).

6. The cause of gastroesophageal reflux disease (GERD) is usually a loosening of the _____ located
   between the esophagus and the stomach.

7. In order to reduce gas bubbles that sometimes cause bloating and discomfort, _____ is sometimes
   added to antacid preparations.

8. Antiemetics are drugs used to treat _____ and _____.

9. Drugs prescribed to induce weight loss are called _____.

MATCHING

For Questions 10–21, match the drug in Column I with its primary class in Column II.

	Column I		**Column II**
10.	_____ Cimetidine (Tagamet)	a.	H$_2$-receptor blocker
11.	_____ Famotidine (Pepcid, Mylanta AP)	b.	Proton-pump inhibitor
12.	_____ Dexamethasone (Decadron)	c.	Antacid
13.	_____ Lansoprazole (Prevacid)	d.	Phenothiazine
14.	_____ Aluminum hydroxide (Amphojel)	e.	Antihistamine
15.	_____ Lorazepam (Ativan)	f.	Antidiarrheal
16.	_____ Ranitidine (Zantac)	g.	Serotonin-receptor blocker
17.	_____ Psyllium muciloid (Metamucil, others)	h.	Laxative
18.	_____ Omeprazole (Prilosec)	i.	Glucocorticoid
19.	_____ Bisacodyl (Dulcolax)	j.	Benzodiazepine
20.	_____ Hydroxyzine (Atarax, Vistaril)		
21.	_____ Prochlorperazine (Compazine)		

MULTIPLE CHOICE

22. Diphenoxylate (Lomotil) is not likely to be abused for its opioid properties because it:

   a. Tastes terrible

   b. Causes diarrhea

   c. Causes impotence and a lack of libido

   d. Contains atropine

23. The nurse would expect the patient to begin vomiting shortly after administering:

   a. Prochlorperazine (Compazine)

   b. Kaopectate

   c. Scopolamine

   d. Syrup of ipecac

24. Some antacids are also marketed as nutritional supplements by claiming to provide daily amounts of which mineral?

   a. Calcium

   b. Sodium

   c. Magnesium

   d. Aluminum

25. Patients receiving _____ are prone to developing peptic ulcers.

    a. Thyroid hormone

    b. Insulin

    c. Glucocorticoids

    d. Estrogens/progestins

26. The most common site for peptic ulcer is the:

    a. Upper stomach

    b. Lower stomach

    c. Duodenum

    d. Large intestine

27. Which of the following serves as a natural defense that helps neutralize stomach acid?

    a. Hydrochloric acid

    b. Bicarbonate ion

    c. Sodium chloride

    d. Potassium chloride

28. The majority of peptic ulcers are caused by:

    a. Infection by *Helicobacter pylori*

    b. Aspirin

    c. Hyposecretion of acid

    d. Hypersecretion of bicarbonate

29. Which of the following is NOT a common sign or symptom of duodenal ulcer?

    a. Gnawing or burning pain in the upper abdomen

    b. Pain that occurs 1–3 hours after a meal

    c. Pain that disappears following ingestion of food

    d. Nausea, vomiting, and pain that occurs during the night

30. Which of the following drug classes is NOT used for peptic ulcer therapy?

    a. H_1-receptor blockers

    b. Antibiotics

    c. Proton-pump inhibitors

    d. Antacids

31. Which class of drugs reduces acid secretion in the stomach by binding irreversibly to the enzyme H^+, K^+–ATPase?

    a. H_2-receptor blockers

    b. Serotonin-receptor blockers

    c. Proton-pump inhibitors

    d. Antacids

32. Which class of drugs acts by neutralizing stomach acid?

    a. H_2-receptor blockers

    b. Serotonin-receptor blockers

    c. Proton-pump inhibitors

    d. Antacids

33. Which class of peptic ulcer medications consists of alkaline combinations of aluminum hydroxide and magnesium hydroxide?

    a. Phenothiazines

    b. Serotonin-receptor blockers

    c. Proton-pump inhibitors

    d. Antacids

34. The nurse would administer amoxicillin (Amoxil) or clarithromycin (Biaxin) for peptic ulcers in order to:

    a. Kill *H. pylori*

    b. Reduce the secretion of acid

    c. Increase the secretion of bicarbonate

    d. Add a gel-like protective mucus over the ulcer

35. Which of the following best describes the mechanism of the action of sucralfate (Carafate)?

    a. Kills *H. pylori*

    b. Adds a gel-like protective mucus over the ulcer

    c. Reduces the secretion of acid

    d. Increases the secretion of bicarbonate

36. Which of the following is NOT a class of drugs used to promote bowel movements?

    a. Opioids

    b. Bulk-forming fiber

    c. Saline/osmotic

    d. Stool softeners/surfactant

37. Which of the following is the most effective class of drugs used to treat diarrhea?

    a. Phenothiazines

    b. Antihistamines

    c. Anticholinergics

    d. Opioids

38. The health care provider may administer which class of drugs to treat motion sickness?

    a. Laxatives

    b. Emetics

    c. Antiemetics

    d. Proton-pump inhibitors

39. In obese patients, sibutramine (Meridia) can induce a weight loss of about _____ over a 12-month period.

    a. 10%

    b. 20%

    c. 30%

    d. 40%

DO YOU REMEMBER?

40. Which of the following would NOT be expected from an overdose of an opioid?

    a. Central nervous system (CNS) depression

    b. Diarrhea

    c. Respiratory depression

    d. Constricted pupils

41. Glucocorticoids are sometimes prescribed for nausea. Which of the following is another indication for this class of drugs?

    a. Peptic ulcers

    b. Asthma

    c. Acute infections

    d. Hypertension

42. Although occasionally used for nausea and vomiting, what is the most common indication for serotonin-receptor blockers?

    a. Schizophrenia

    b. Epilepsy

    c. Attention deficit disorder (ADD)/attention deficit–hyperactivity disorder (ADHD)

    d. Depression

43. Mr. H is receiving an HMG-CoA reductase inhibitor. He is most likely being treated for:

    a. High lipid levels in the blood

    b. Stroke

    c. Schizophrenia

    d. Hypertension

44. Ms. L has just returned from South America, where she contracted traveler's diarrhea due to parasites in the water. Which drug would be most effective against these protozoans?

    a. Ciprofloxacin (Cipro)

    b. Cloxacillin (Cloxapen)

    c. Metronidazole (Flagyl)

    d. Ceftizoxime (Cefizox)

CASE STUDY APPLICATIONS

45. Mr. D enters your clinic with a complaint of severe upper abdominal pain that occurs mostly in the evening hours. It is relieved by food, although he vomits his meals several times each week. He has a history of peptic ulcers and alcohol abuse, and he claims his smoking has been reduced to two packs per week. Laboratory results reveal blood in his stools. He is taking no drugs, other than Rolaids, for his indigestion. The physician suspects peptic ulcer disease.

    a. Are Mr. D's symptoms characteristic of duodenal or gastric ulcers?

    b. What lifestyle changes may be contributing to Mr. D's condition?

    c. What are the pharmacotherapeutic options for Mr. D?

46. Ms. V is an elderly patient who comes to your clinic complaining of fullness in her abdomen and constipation. Ms. V is mostly homebound due to severe arthritis and a hip fracture last year. She claims that her diet is normal, although her son who accompanied her disagrees. Her son states that Ms. V eats only one meal per day, consisting usually of white bread and turkey slices. He is also concerned that his mother is taking Ex-Lax every day. Ms. V's physician finds her to be in otherwise good health for her age and medical history.

    a. Are there lifestyle changes that may be contributing to Ms. V's complaints?

    b. What are some therapeutic options available for Ms. V?

CHAPTER 30

VITAMINS, MINERALS, AND NUTRITIONAL SUPPLEMENTS

LEARNING OUTCOMES

To view the objectives, please refer to the textbook or
MyNursingKit™ at www.mynursingkit.com.

TRUE/FALSE

For Questions 1–7, choose T for true or F for false.

T F 1. The body can synthesize small amounts of all the water-
and fat-soluble vitamins.

T F 2. Iodine is a mineral important to the health of the thyroid
gland.

T F 3. Water-soluble vitamins cannot be stored by the body and must be ingested daily.

T F 4. Enteral nutrition includes products delivered through intravenous feeding.

T F 5. Because macrominerals are needed daily in large amounts, most patients require mineral supplements.

T F 6. Vitamin B_{12} is not synthesized by either plants or animals; only bacteria can make this vitamin.

T F 7. With the exception of vitamins A and D, it is not harmful for most patients to consume two to three time
the recommended daily allowance (RDA) of vitamins.

FILL IN THE BLANK

From the text, find the correct word(s) to complete the statement(s).

8. Vitamin _____ is an antidote to overdose with the anticoagulant warfarin (Coumadin).

9. The most common nutritional deficiency in the world is _____.

10. If they are taken in excessive amounts, _____-soluble vitamins may result in hypervitaminosis.

11. After red blood cells become worn out and die, nearly all of the iron in their hemoglobin is _____

MATCHING

For Questions 12–17, match the vitamin in Column I with its classification in Column II.

Column I	Column II
12. _____ Vitamin C	a. Water soluble
13. _____ Vitamin B complex	b. Fat soluble
14. _____ Vitamin A	
15. _____ Vitamin D	
16. _____ Vitamin E	
17. _____ Vitamin K	

MULTIPLE CHOICE

18. Total parenteral nutrition often involves the administration of:

    a. Amino acids

    b. Lipids

    c. Carbohydrates

    d. All of the above

19. The RDA represents the:

    a. Minimum amount of vitamin or mineral needed to prevent a deficiency in a healthy adult

    b. Maximum amount of vitamin or mineral needed to prevent a deficiency in a healthy adult

    c. Minimum amount of vitamin or mineral needed to prevent a deficiency in someone who is pregnant or has special nutritional needs

    d. Maximum amount of vitamin or mineral needed to prevent a deficiency in someone who is pregnant or has special nutritional needs

20. Which of the following vitamins would be the most hazardous to ingest in amounts in excess of the RDA?

    a. A

    b. B complex

    c. C

    d. E

21. Which of the following is NOT a B vitamin?

    a. Niacin

    b. Cobalamin

    c. Biotin

    d. Pyridoxine

22. Which of the following is a common cause of vitamin deficiency in the United States?

    a. Drug therapy with antibiotics

    b. Ingestion of excess cholesterol

    c. Opioid addiction

    d. Alcoholism

23. Cyanocobalamin is a purified form of vitamin:

    a. C

    b. B_{12}

    c. K

    d. E

24. Alcohol abuse is the most common cause of _____ deficiency in the United States.

    a. Thiamine

    b. Vitamin B_{12}

    c. Iron

    d. Potassium

25. The most common cause of vitamin B_{12} deficiency is lack of:

    a. Green leafy vegetables in the diet

    b. Iron in the diet

    c. Intrinsic factor

    d. Meat in the diet

26. Which of the following is a major mineral?

    a. Magnesium

    b. Molybdenum

    c. Copper

    d. Fluoride

27. Which of the following is a trace mineral?

    a. Sulfur

    b. Phosphorus

    c. Calcium

    d. Selenium

28. Ferrous sulfate (Ferralyn) is a form of:

    a. Vitamin B_{12}

    b. Copper

    c. Iron

    d. Sodium

29. Pernicious or megaloblastic anemia is due to a deficiency of:

    a. Red blood cells

    b. Iron

    c. Macrominerals

    d. Vitamin B_{12}

30. Sixty to eighty percent of all iron in the body is associated with:

    a. Hemoglobin

    b. Hemosiderin

    c. Sulfur

    d. Vitamin B_{12}

31. A patient is taking iron supplements. The nurse would teach this patient that the most common side effects of iron therapy relate to which body system?

    a. Cardiovascular

    b. Digestive

    c. Urinary

    d. Nervous

32. The nurse should recommend to patients that iron supplements be administered:

    a. With milk

    b. 1 hour before or 2 hours after a meal

    c. With a meal

    d. In the morning, on awakening

33. Ms. T is an 80-year-old patient who is being treated for osteoporosis. For this condition, the nurse should recommend that Ms. T receive plenty of:

    a. Vitamin A

    b. Sodium

    c. Calcium

    d. Iodide

34. A patient is likely to receive total parenteral nutrition (TPN) for which of the following conditions?

    a. Major surgery

    b. Bowel obstruction

    c. Supplemental oral intake

    d. Difficulty swallowing

DO YOU REMEMBER?

35. Certain diuretics are sometimes prescribed to prevent excess loss of:

    a. Chloride

    b. Sodium

    c. Potassium

    d. Iron

36. An unlabeled use of cyanocobalamin is to treat toxicity associated with the administration of sodium nitroprusside. The health care provider would most likely administer sodium nitroprusside for:

    a. Shock

    b. Hypertensive crisis

    c. An agitated patient with schizophrenia

    d. Status epilepticus

37. Ferrous sulfate has a tendency to cause constipation in certain patients. The nurse might recommend which of the following to counteract this side effect?

    a. Bismuth salts (Pepto-Bismol)

    b. Prochlorperazine (Compazine)

    c. Mylanta

    d. Docusate (Surfak)

38. Ms. C is taking tacrine (Cognex) 10 mg qid. It is likely that Ms. C has:

    a. Alzheimer's disease

    b. Insomnia

    c. Epilepsy

    d. Parkinson's disease

39. Ms. L is receiving foscarnet (Foscavir) for a herpes-simplex viral infection. The nurse might recommend which inexpensive antacid to prevent the hypocalcemia that commonly occurs with this antiviral?

    a. Tums

    b. Maalox

    c. Amphojel

    d. Riopan

CASE STUDY APPLICATION

40. As a home health care provider, you are interviewing Mr. N, an elderly patient, in his home to obtain a nutritional assessment. The patient does not take vitamin or mineral supplements. He claims that they are too expensive and he has read that a normal diet provides all the nutrients needed. Further, Mr. N claims to eat plenty of "normal" food. During the assessment, it is determined that the patient does, indeed, have a varied diet, although his intake is slightly less than average for a man of his age.

   a. Is Mr. N correct when he states that all necessary nutrients can be obtained through a "normal" diet? How would you respond?

   b. During your assessment, what data, other than food intake, would be important to collect in order to determine if Mr. N might benefit from vitamin or mineral supplementation?

   c. Why are elderly patients more at risk for vitamin deficiency disorders than younger patients?

CHAPTER 31

DRUGS FOR ENDOCRINE DISORDERS

LEARNING OUTCOMES

To view the objectives, please refer to the textbook or MyNursingKit™ at www.mynursingkit.com.

TRUE/FALSE

For Questions 1–8, choose T for true or F for false.

T F 1. When hormones are administered as replacement therapy, the body's negative feedback mechanism is inactivated.

T F 2. The endocrine structure in the brain that is responsible for secreting releasing factors is the pituitary gland.

T F 3. With type 2 diabetes mellitus, the pancreas is unable to secrete insulin and, therefore, insulin therapy is usually required.

T F 4. The treatment goal with insulin therapy is to maintain blood glucose levels within strict, normal limits.

T F 5. A primary function of the thyroid gland is to control basal metabolic rate.

T F 6. Levothyroxine (Synthroid) is a synthetic form of thyroxine (T_4) used for replacement therapy in patients with low thyroid function.

T F 7. Significant adverse effects are not usually a problem during long-term therapy with glucocorticoids.

T F 8. Of the many different hormones secreted by the pituitary and hypothalamus, only a few are used for drug therapy.

FILL IN THE BLANK

From the text, find the correct word(s) to complete the statement(s).

9. _____ are chemical messengers released in response to a change in the body's internal environment.

10. Releasing hormones signal the _____ to release the hormone necessary to create a desired effect in the body.

11. When administering antidiuretic hormones, the nurse should carefully assess fluid and _____ balance.

12. Vasopressin injection (Pitressin) should never be administered by the _____ route.

13. Prior to administration of levothyroxine (Synthroid), the nurse should thoroughly assess the patient's _____ system.

14. Graves' disease may cause tachycardia, weight loss, elevated body temperature, and _____.

15. Propylthiouracil (PTU) may cause gastrointestinal (GI) distress and should be administered _____ meals.

16. The nurse must be aware that glucocorticoids increase the patient's susceptibility to _____.

17. Juvenile-onset diabetes is called _____; age-onset diabetes is referred to as _____.

18. A class of drugs prescribed after diet and exercise have failed to bring blood glucose levels to within normal limits is _____.

19. In type 2 diabetes mellitus, insulin receptors in the target tissues have become _____ to the hormone.

20. The treatment goal with insulin therapy is to maintain _____ levels within strict, normal limits.

21. Acute pancreatitis may occur suddenly and most commonly exhibits symptoms of _____.

22. _____ elevates the protein content of pancreatic juices and contributes to the formation of stones, which may block pancreatic ducts.

MATCHING

For Questions 23–27, match the specific disease in Column I with its related concept in Column II.

Column I	Column II
23. _____ Cushing's syndrome	a. Thyroid hormone (Synthroid)
24. _____ Adrenal cortex hyposecretion	b. Vasopressin (Pitressin)
25. _____ Graves' disease	c. Linked to use of glucocorticoid medication
26. _____ Myxedema (adults) and cretinism (children)	d. Glucocorticoid release from tissue
27. _____ Diabetes insipidus	e. Propylthiouracil (PTU)

For Questions 28–30, match the drug in Column I with its class in Column II.

Column I	Column II
28. _____ Prednisone (Deltasone, others)	a. Thyroid medication
29. _____ Liotrix (Euthroid, others)	b. Antithyroid medication
30. _____ Methimazole (Tapazole)	c. Glucocorticoid

For Questions 31–33, match the specific disease in Column I with the drug therapy in Column II.

Column I	Column II
31. _____ Type 1 diabetes mellitus	a. Pancrelipase (Lipancreatin)
32. _____ Type 2 diabetes mellitus	b. Regular insulin (Humulin R)
33. _____ Chronic pancreatitis	c. Glipizide (Glucotrol)

For Questions 34–36, match the drug in Column I with its class in Column II.

Column I	Column II
34. _____ Pancrelipase (Lipancreatin)	a. Hypoglycemics
35. _____ Regular insulin (Humulin R)	b. Insulin
36. _____ Glipizide (Glucotrol)	c. Pancreatic enzyme replacement

MULTIPLE CHOICE

37. The nurse is monitoring a patient's laboratory tests and notices a rise in parathyroid hormone (PTH). Which of the following laboratory values may also occur in this patient?

   a. Increased blood glucose

   b. Decreased blood glucose

   c. Decreased serum calcium

   d. Increased serum calcium

38. The nurse understands that negative feedback ensures endocrine homeostasis by doing which of the following?

   a. Stimulating the release of a secondary hormone

   b. Stimulating the release of a primary hormone

   c. Inhibiting the action of a secondary hormone

   d. Inhibiting the action of a primary hormone

39. The nurse is caring for a patient who is receiving hormone replacement therapy (HRT). Which of the following is NOT an example of HRT?

   a. Thyroid hormone after thyroidectomy

   b. Insulin for a patient whose pancreas is not functioning

   c. Testosterone for breast cancer

   d. Adrenal cortex dysfunction

40. Which of the following hormones is NOT released from the anterior pituitary gland?

   a. Thyroid-stimulating hormone (TSH)

   b. Antidiuretic hormone (ADH)

   c. Growth hormone

   d. Adrenocorticotropic hormone (ACTH)

41. A patient receiving levothyroxine (Synthroid) would be expected to experience which of the following adverse metabolic effects?

    a. Loss of weight

    b. Lack of energy

    c. Reduced pulse rate

    d. Reduced body temperature

42. It is important that the nurse teach female patients that long-term use of levothyroxine (Synthroid) may be associated with which of the following symptoms?

    a. Osteoporosis

    b. Decreased white blood cell count

    c. Weight gain

    d. Decreased incidence of insomnia

43. The nurse would most likely administer antithyroid medications to patients with which of the following symptoms?

    a. Dysrhythmia

    b. Weight loss

    c. Reduced activity

    d. Anemia

44. Which of the following hormones will ultimately result in the release of glucocorticoids from the adrenal glands?

    a. Corticotropin releasing factor (CRF)

    b. ACTH

    c. Falling levels of cortisol

    d. All of the above

45. Which of the following drugs is often administered by alternate-day dosing and requires the nurse to provide specific patient teaching?

    a. Thyroid hormone

    b. Antithyroid therapy

    c. Corticosteroids

    d. Insulin

46. In caring for a patient with Cushing's syndrome, the nurse understands that this disorder is associated with which of the following hormones?

    a. Mineralocorticoids

    b. Glucocorticoids

    c. Androgens

    d. ADH

47. The nurse should observe for which of the following adverse effects of hydrocortisone (Cortef, Hydrocortone) therapy?

    a. Asthma

    b. Rhinitis

    c. Nausea

    d. Mood and personality changes

48. Which of the following corticosteroids has mineralocorticoid activity?

    a. Hydrocortisone (Cortef, Hydrocortone)

    b. Methylprednisolone (Solu-Medrol, Medrol)

    c. Prednisolone (Delta-Cortef)

    d. Prednisone (Deltasone, others)

49. A deficiency of growth hormone will result in which of the following?

    a. Dwarfism

    b. Diabetes insipidus

    c. Urinary retention

    d. Mental impairment

50. Vasopressin (Pitressin) is prescribed for which of the following primary symptoms?

    a. Altered metabolism

    b. Polyuria

    c. Inflammation

    d. Altered glucose blood levels

51. Which of the following stimulates the pancreas to secrete insulin?

    a. Hyperglycemia

    b. Hypoglycemia

    c. Glucagon

    d. Ketoacids

52. While taking a health history, the nurse should recognize that which of the following is NOT a short-term sign of type 1 diabetes mellitus?

    a. Polyuria

    b. Polyphagia

    c. Acidosis

    d. Polydipsia

53. When giving insulin, the nurse knows that the most common route of administration is which of the following?

    a. Oral

    b. Intradermal

    c. Subcutaneous

    d. Intramuscular

54. When planning follow-up care, the nurse should know that which of the following is a longer-acting form of insulin?

    a. Insulin lispro (Humalog)

    b. Insulin, isophane (Humulin N, others)

    c. Insulin lente (Humulin L, Novolin L, others)

    d. Insulin ultralente (Humulin U, Ultralente)

55. Which of the following adverse effects does the nurse recognize when too much insulin has been administered?

    a. Hypoglycemia

    b. Tachycardia

    c. Convulsions

    d. All of the above

56. When giving oral hypoglycemics, the nurse expects which of the following actions to occur?

    a. The pancreas is stimulated to secrete more insulin.

    b. Insulin receptors become more sensitive to target tissues.

    c. The liver is inhibited from releasing glucose.

    d. Both a and b are correct.

57. Which of the following administration techniques applies to pancrelipase (Ultrase)?

    a. Crush enteric-coated tablets.

    b. Swallow enteric-coated tablets.

    c. Give 4 hours following meals.

    d. Give slow IV push.

58. During oral hypoglycemic therapy, the nurse should assess for which symptoms related to abnormalities in liver function?

    a. Yellowed skin, pale stools, dark urine

    b. Pink skin, light brown stools, yellow urine

    c. Pale skin, red-tinged stools, amber urine

    d. Red skin, dark stools, clear urine

59. If injections sites are not rotated regularly, the patient with diabetes may suffer from which of the following?

    a. Petechiae

    b. Lipodystrophy

    c. Hematoma

    d. Pustules

60. Which of the following nursing diagnoses is NOT appropriate for the patient receiving insulin therapy?

    a. Risk for injury

    b. Risk for imbalanced nutrition

    c. Risk for role confusion

    d. Risk for infection

61. When considering glucose regulation in the body, which of the following components of homeostasis would be restored following insulin therapy?

    a. Sensor (senses glucose in the bloodstream)

    b. Control center (determines the set point for glucose levels in the bloodstream)

    c. Effector (responds to the increased levels of glucose in the bloodstream)

    d. Receptor (produces a response at the site of glucose action)

DO YOU REMEMBER?

62. Which of the following will change during thyroid therapy if only heart rate increases?

    a. Dysrhythmia

    b. Peripheral vascular resistance

    c. Cardiac output

    d. Stroke volume

63. Cholestyramine (Questran) will decrease the absorption of levothyroxine (Synthroid) if given at the same time. Patients take cholestyramine for what type of disorders?

    a. Hypertension

    b. High blood cholesterol level

    c. Peptic ulcer

    d. Weight gain

64. Fluconazole (Diflucan) and other azole drugs are indicated for which of the following?

    a. Fungal infection

    b. Malaria

    c. Diarrhea

    d. Constipation

65. Which vitamin is considered to be an antidote for overdoses of warfarin (Coumadin)?

    a. A

    b. B_2

    c. B_{12}

    d. K

66. A drug's trade name is assigned by which of the following?

    a. Physician

    b. Pharmacist

    c. Drug manufacturer

    d. Food and Drug Administration (FDA)

67. A patient is prescribed pancrelipase (Ultrase) and takes iron supplements. The nurse is aware that taking these drugs together may do which of the following?

    a. Increase iron absorption

    b. Decrease iron absorption

    c. Increase zymase absorption

    d. Decrease zymase absorption

68. Prior to administration of medications for pancreatitis, assessing for alcohol abuse is necessary because alcohol can do which of the following?

    a. Contribute to stone formation and pancreatic inflammation

    b. Cause inhibition of gastric secretions

    c. Enhance lung expansion

    d. Elevate blood pH

69. Why must the nurse instruct a patient receiving glipizide (Glucotrol XL) to avoid crushing or chewing the tablets?

    a. The patient may choke.

    b. The effectiveness of the medication would be hindered.

    c. It would cause blood glucose levels to rise too rapidly.

    d. Irritation of the oral mucosa may occur.

70. Monoamine oxidase (MAO) inhibitors may potentiate hypoglycemic effects when used with which of the following drugs?

    a. Insulin

    b. Dextrothyroxine

    c. Corticosteroids

    d. Epinephrine

CASE STUDY APPLICATIONS

71. Ms. Z has diabetes and is a candidate for thyroid therapy because of her hypothyroid disorder. Examples of the medications she might take include levothyroxine sodium (Synthroid, others), liothyronine sodium (Cytomel), and liotrix (Euthroid, others).

    a. In planning proper care, what complications of using these drugs simultaneously would the nurse consider?

    b. What nursing interventions would be appropriate?

72. Mr. D, age 35, is diagnosed with Graves' disease. He wants to know how his new medication, propylthiouracil (PTU), will impact his life.

    a. List the important patient teaching related to PTU.

    b. Describe nursing interventions that will assist this patient in adjusting to his medication regimen.

73. Mr. D is 70 years old and has type 2 diabetes mellitus. You are performing an initial assessment.

    a. Which kind of diabetic therapy would he likely require?

    b. Explain the patient teaching needed for Mr. D, including difficulties that may arise.

74. The nurse is planning discharge teaching for Mr. C, a patient recently diagnosed with chronic pancreatitis. He lives alone, has little to no income, and does not have transportation.

    a. What important points should the nurse include in discharge planning?

    b. What data from the patient's social history will take special analysis when planning care?

75. Mr. R lives within 2 miles of a nuclear power plant. He comes to the doctor's office to request "the pills that make you immune to radiation sickness." Because you are aware that nurses play a key role in educating the public regarding bioterrorism, you have developed a standard care plan regarding nuclear disaster education for patients who live near the power plant.

    a. What patient teaching should you give to Mr. R regarding potassium iodide?

    b. In evaluating Mr. R's understanding of the information he has been given, you ask him to explain why potassium iodide is effective in preventing thyroid cancer after radiation exposure. What should be his answer?

CHAPTER 32

DRUGS FOR DISORDERS AND CONDITIONS OF THE REPRODUCTIVE SYSTEM

LEARNING OUTCOMES

To view the objectives, please refer to the textbook or MyNursingKit™ at www.mynursingkit.com.

TRUE/FALSE

For Questions 1–14, choose T for true or F for false.

T F 1. *Estrogen* is actually a generic term for three different sex hormones named estradiol, estrone, and estriol.

T F 2. The cyclic secretion of estrogen and progesterone in women is similar to the secretion of testosterone in men.

T F 3. The most common progestin used in oral contraceptives is ethinyl estradiol.

T F 4. Triphasil is an oral contraceptive containing both ethinyl estradiol and norgestrel.

T F 5. When used appropriately, oral contraceptives are nearly 100% effective.

T F 6. The progestin-only oral contraceptive prevents pregnancy primarily by preventing ovulation.

T F 7. Monophasic formulations of oral contraception contain both an estrogen and a progestin.

T F 8. Estrogen is rarely used to treat prostate cancer.

T F 9. Progestins are occasionally prescribed for the treatment of metastatic endometrial carcinoma.

T F 10. Androgens are sex hormones secreted only by male patients.

T F 11. Tocolytics are drugs used to stimulate uterine contractions.

T F 12. Oxytocin (Pitocin) may be infused to stimulate contractions of the uterus during labor and delivery.

T F 13. Testosterone (Andro) is a category X drug and should not be taken if pregnancy is suspected or confirmed.

T F 14. There is currently no drug therapy available to treat benign enlargement of the prostate.

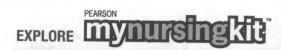

FILL IN THE BLANK

From the text, find the correct word(s) to complete the statement(s).

15. _____ is the hormone that regulates sperm or egg production; _____ in women triggers the release of the egg, a process known as ovulation.

16. The permanent cessation of menses, caused by lack of estrogen secretion by the ovaries, is _____.

17. The class of drugs called _____ exerts positive metabolic effects in postmenopausal women, including an increase in bone mass and a reduction in low-density lipoprotein (LDL) cholesterol.

18. The absence of menstruation is called _____.

19. Hormones called _____ are often prescribed for dysfunctional uterine bleeding.

20. The anterior pituitary hormone called _____ increases the synthesis of milk within the mammary glands; the posterior pituitary hormone called _____ causes milk to be ejected.

21. _____ are testosterone-like compounds with hormonal activity.

22. A side effect of testosterone therapy in female patients is the appearance of masculine characteristics, or _____.

23. The oral medication first approved for erectile dysfunction, in 1998, was _____.

24. _____ is an enlargement of the prostate gland that occurs mostly in men of advanced age.

MATCHING

For Questions 25–29, match the medication in Column I with its drug classification in Column II.

Column I	Column II
25. _____ Norethindrone (Micronor)	a. Estrogen
26. _____ Estradiol valerate (Delestrogen)	b. Progestin
27. _____ Terbutaline sulfate (Brethine)	c. Uterine stimulant
28. _____ Danazol (Danocrine)	d. Tocolytic
29. _____ Misoprostol (Cytotec)	e. Androgen

For Questions 30–35, match the drug classification in Column I with its indication in Column II. Use each answer only once.

Column I	Column II
30. _____ Progestins	a. Delayed puberty in men and breast cancer
31. _____ Estrogens	b. Dysfunctional uterine bleeding
32. _____ Androgens	c. Replacement therapy in women and prostate cancer in men
33. _____ Oral contraceptives	d. Premature labor
34. _____ Oxytocin	e. Labor induction
35. _____ Tocolytics	f. Prevention conception

MULTIPLE CHOICE

36. Which of the following oral contraceptives is a triphasic type?

    a. Alesse

    b. Lo/Ovral

    c. Ortho-Cyclin

    d. Ortho-Novum

37. Which of the following potential consequences of estrogen loss are related to postmenopausal conditions?

    a. Insomnia

    b. Sexual disinterest

    c. Mood disturbances

    d. Osteoporosis

38. Which of the following medications is used to treat endometriosis?

    a. Estropipate (Ogen)

    b. Ethinyl estradiol (Ethinyl, Feminone)

    c. Estradiol (Estraderm, Estrace)

    d. Norethindrone acetate

39. Which of the following uterine stimulants may also be used for short-term treatment of gastric ulcers?

    a. Oxytocin (Pitocin, Syntocinon)

    b. Misoprostol (Cytotec)

    c. Dinoprostone (Cervidil)

    d. Methylergonovine maleate (Methergine)

40. Which of the following medications would NOT be used to treat postpartum breast engorgement?

    a. Medroxyprogesterone (Provera, Cycrin)

    b. Estradiol (Estraderm, Estrace)

    c. Testosterone (Andro 100)

    d. Fluoxymesterone (Halotestin)

41. Which of the following medications may be used as an anticonvulsant in pre-eclampsia?

    a. Oxytocin (Pitocin)

    b. Magnesium sulfate

    c. Terbutaline sulfate (Brethine)

    d. Ritodrine hydrochloride (Yutopar)

42. Which class of medications can decrease the effectiveness of oral contraceptives?

    a. Antibiotics

    b. Antineoplastics

    c. Calcium channel blockers

    d. Antihypertensives

43. Which of the following releases steroid hormones such as estrogen and androgens?

    a. Pituitary gland

    b. Pancreas

    c. Adrenal gland

    d. Hypothalamus

44. Erectile dysfunction may be successfully treated with:

    a. Testosterone (Andro 100)

    b. Sildenafil (Viagra)

    c. Finasteride (Proscar)

    d. Doxazocin (Cardura)

45. Which of the following diseases are often associated with erectile dysfunction?

    a. Diabetes

    b. Hypertension

    c. Benign prostatic hyperplasia (BPH)

    d. a and b

46. Which of the following oral contraceptives acts by producing a thick cervical mucus?

    a. Progesterone micronized (Prometrium)

    b. Estradiol (Estraderm, Estrace)

    c. Danazol (Danocrine)

    d. Nandrolone phenproprionate (Durabolin, Hybolin)

47. Which of the following medications is used for termination of early pregnancy?

    a. Estropipate (Ogen)

    b. Fluoxymesterone (Halotestin)

    c. Mifepristone (RU 486)

    d. Ritodrine hydrochloride (Yutopar)

48. Which of the following is NOT a benefit of conjugated estrogens and progestins therapy?

    a. Lowered risk of colon cancer

    b. Reduction in LDL cholesterol

    c. Weight loss

    d. Increase in bone mass

49. The function of natural progesterone is to:

   a. Build up the lining of the uterus

   b. Prevent ovulation

   c. Prepare the uterus for implantation of the embryo

   d. Induce menstrual bleeding

50. Oral contraceptives are contraindicated in patients with which of the following disorders?

   a. Hypertension

   b. Hyperglycemia

   c. Potential for blood clots and stroke

   d. Depression

51. One of the adverse effects of anabolic steroids is:

   a. Liver damage

   b. The appearance of masculine characteristics

   c. Muscle weakness

   d. Cardiovascular disease

DO YOU REMEMBER?

52. Stress often has an effect on the release of hormones. Which of the following nervous system components would activate hormonal release at the level of the hypothalamus and adrenal glands?

   a. Somatic nervous system

   b. Sympathetic nervous system

   c. Central nervous system

   d. Sensory nervous system

53. Glucocorticoids would produce an effect at which of the following target receptor locations?

   a. Plasma membrane of the target cell

   b. Cytoplasm of the target cell

   c. Nucleus of the target cell

   d. Cellular component other than the nucleus

54. Cimetidine (Tagamet) is sometimes given to patients who are taking glucocorticoids in order to prevent:

   a. Hypertension

   b. Constipation

   c. Thromboembolic disease

   d. Peptic ulcer disease

55. Where would you most likely find the barbiturate thiopental sodium (Pentothal) in use?

    a. Coronary care unit

    b. Sleep disorder clinic

    c. Cancer clinic

    d. Surgical suite

56. Interferon alpha-2a is classified as a(n):

    a. Alkylating agent

    b. Biologic response modifier

    c. Hormone

    d. Coagulation modifier

CASE STUDY APPLICATIONS

57. Ms. M, age 50, is concerned about the unpleasant effects accompanying menopause. Her last menstrual period was several months ago, and she is beginning to experience hot flashes, night sweats, nervousness, and insomnia. The nurse suggests hormone replacement therapy (HRT). Ms. M states that she knows nothing about HRT.

    a. What nursing diagnosis is appropriate for Ms. M? State the expected outcome for this nursing diagnosis.

    b. State the patient teaching necessary to assist Ms. M in achieving the expected outcome.

58. Mrs. E, a primigravida who is 30 weeks pregnant, is in labor. Following rupture of membranes, she is receiving oxytocin IV.

    a. What assessment data are necessary for the nurse to gather to monitor for adverse effects?

    b. List nursing actions related to this medication.

59. Mr. E, a 62-year-old patient, is receiving finasteride (Proscar) due to an enlarged prostate. He asks the nurse how he will know if the medication is working and when he can stop taking it.

    a. List the nursing interventions and patient teaching appropriate for Mr. E.

    b. State specifically how the nurse will evaluate medication effectiveness.

60. Mr. S, a 38-year-old married man, has been diagnosed with low testosterone levels. Mr. S has type 1 diabetes and prides himself in his knowledge of herb use related to health.

    a. What assessment data are important for the nurse to obtain before Mr. S begins androgen therapy?

    b. What nursing interventions and patient education are appropriate for Mr. S related to his diabetes?

CHAPTER 33

DRUGS FOR BONE
AND JOINT DISORDERS

LEARNING OUTCOMES

To view the objectives, please refer to the textbook or
MyNursingKit™ at www.mynursingkit.com.

TRUE/FALSE

For Questions 1–7, choose T for true or F for false.

T F 1. Calcifediol is the active form of vitamin D.

T F 2. Bone deposition is the process whereby bone is broken
          down into smaller mineral components.

T F 3. Parathyroid hormone stimulates the formation of calcitriol
          within the kidneys.

T F 4. Osteomalacia is caused by excessive amounts of vitamin D and calcium in the body.

T F 5. When estrogen blood levels are low, bones become weak and fragile, which can result in osteoporosis.

T F 6. Weak and fragile bones are improved by drugs that inhibit bone resorption.

T F 7. Osteoarthritis is sometimes called noninflammatory-type arthritis because it is not accompanied
          by inflammation.

FILL IN THE BLANK

From the text, find the correct word(s) to complete the statement(s).

8. Disorders associated with _____ are some of the most difficult conditions to treat because of the
   mechanisms underlying them.

9. Movement disorders span the _____, _____, _____, and
   _____ body systems.

10. One of the most important minerals in the body responsible for bone formation is _____.

 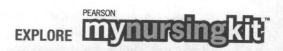

11. Calcium levels in the bloodstream are controlled by two endocrine glands, the _____ glands and the _____ gland.

12. Calcium disorders are often related to _____ disorders.

13. Osteomalacia, referred to as _____ in children, is a disorder characterized by the softening of bones without alteration of basic bone structure.

14. Two important disorders characterized by weak and fragile bones are _____ and _____.

15. The hormone responsible for bone resorption is _____; the hormone responsible for bone deposition is _____.

16. Cholecalciferol is converted to an intermediate vitamin form called _____; this intermediate form is transported to the kidneys, where enzymes transform it into _____, an active form of vitamin D.

17. The two major forms of calcium used in pharmacotherapy are _____ and _____.

18. _____ is a class of drugs that provide the same protection against uterine or breast cancer as progesterone in estrogen replacement therapy (ERT).

19. A class of drugs called _____ is chemically similar to natural biphosphates found in body tissues.

20. Two drug therapies for Paget's disease are _____ and _____.

21. _____ treat rheumatoid arthritis by suppressing autoimmunity.

22. Drugs preventing the accumulation of uric acid in the bloodstream or joint cavities are called _____.

MATCHING

For Questions 23–29, match the drug in Column I with its classification in Column II.

Column I	**Column II**
23. _____ Calcitriol (Calcijex, Rocaltrol)	a. Calcium supplement
24. _____ Calcium carbonate (BioCal)	b. Vitamin D therapy
25. _____ Allopurinol (Lopurin, Zyloprim)	c. Inhibitor of bone resorption
26. _____ Etidronate disodium (Didronel)	d. Disease-modifying drug
27. _____ Aurothioglucose (Gold Thioglucose, Solganal)	e. Uric acid inhibitor
28. _____ Colchicine	
29. _____ Alendronate (Fosamax)	

For Questions 30–34 match the indication in Column I with its drug in Column II.

Column I

30. _____ Osteomalacia, rickets, and hypocalcemia

31. _____ Osteoporosis, Paget's disease

32. _____ Gouty arthritis

33. _____ Rheumatoid arthritis

34. _____ Osteoarthritis

Column II

a. Alendronate sodium (Fosamax)

b. Probenecid (Benemid)

c. Ergocalciferol (Deltalin, Calciferol)

d. Hydroxychloroquine sulfate (Plaquenil Sulfate)

e. Sodium hyaluronate (Hyalgan)

MULTIPLE CHOICE

35. Which of the following statements regarding calcium in the body is false?

   a. When concentrations are too high, sodium permeability decreases across cell membranes.

   b. When concentrations are too low, cell membranes become hyperexcitable.

   c. Calcium must be present for the body to form vitamin D.

   d. Calcium is important for body processes such as blood coagulation and muscle contraction.

36. Diseases and conditions of calcium and vitamin D metabolism include all of the following EXCEPT:

   a. Osteomalacia

   b. Rheumatoid arthritis

   c. Osteoporosis

   d. Paget's disease

37. Possible etiologies of hypocalcemia include all of the following EXCEPT:

   a. Hyposecretion of parathyroid hormone

   b. Digestive-related malabsorption disorders

   c. Lack of adequate intake of calcium-containing foods

   d. Paget's disease

38. As a health care worker, you are helping your elderly patient, who has osteoporosis, to pick her menu. Which of the following choices would be LEAST useful in helping her maintain adequate calcium intake?

   a. Carton of milk for breakfast

   b. Salmon croquette for dinner

   c. Turnip greens for dinner

   d. Baked potato for lunch

39. Calcium gluconate is contraindicated in patients with all of the following conditions EXCEPT:

    a. Osteomalacia

    b. Digitalis toxicity

    c. Kidney stones

    d. Cardiac dysrhythmias

40. Patient teaching regarding vitamin D therapy includes all of the following EXCEPT:

    a. Take exactly as directed; it can become toxic if taken in excess quantities.

    b. Avoid alcohol and other hepatotoxic drugs.

    c. Avoid sunlight exposure due to susceptibility to sunburn.

    d. Do not start a low-fat diet unless first discussed with the nurse.

41. All of the following are risks factors for osteoporosis EXCEPT:

    a. Anorexia nervosa

    b. Use of ERT

    c. High alcohol or caffeine consumption

    d. Advancing age in women

42. Which of the following statements regarding calcitonin is false?

    a. It is obtained from salmon.

    b. It is currently available only in oral form.

    c. It increases bone density and reduces the incidence of vertebral fractures.

    d. It is indicated for Paget's disease and hypercalcemia.

43. Selective estrogen receptor modulators (SERMs) are contraindicated in patients with all of the following conditions EXCEPT:

    a. Thromboembolism

    b. Pregnancy or lactation

    c. Hormone replacement

    d. Postmenopause

44. Which of the following is NOT a symptom of osteomalacia and/or rickets?

    a. Hypocalcemia

    b. Convulsions

    c. Muscle weakness

    d. Bowlegs and a pigeon breast

45. After analgesic and anti-inflammatory drugs have been tried, which of the following therapies may be used to alter the course of rheumatoid arthritis progression?

    a. Bisphosphonates

    b. Calcitonin therapy

    c. Disease-modifying drugs

    d. Uric acid inhibitors

46. Which of the following gout medications is used for an acute attack and may cause gastric upset?

    a. Colchicine

    b. Allopurinol (Lopurin)

    c. Penicillamine (Cuprimine, Depen)

    d. Sulfasalazine (Azulfidine)

47. Sodium hyaluronate (Hyalgan) is a new therapy for patients with moderate osteoarthritis. Which of the following statements about this drug is false?

    a. It is injected directly into the knee joint.

    b. It coats the articulating cartilage surface.

    c. Patients should avoid strenuous activity for 48 hours after it is administered.

    d. It is used prior to treatments with COX-2 inhibitors and nonsteroidal anti-inflammatory drugs (NSAIDs).

48. Which of the following patients is LEAST likely to present with gout?

    a. Pacific Islander

    b. Man

    c. Woman

    d. Patient using a thiazide diuretic

DO YOU REMEMBER?

49. What is the neurotransmitter for skeletal muscle contraction?

    a. Acetylcholine

    b. Serotonin

    c. Norepinephrine

    d. Epinephrine

50. Which normal physiologic action other than muscle contraction depends on calcium?

    a. Relaxation of blood vessels

    b. Termination of neurotransmitter action

    c. Transmission of a pain impulse

    d. Blood coagulation

51. Vitamin D can be synthesized from which of the following chemicals?

    a. Triglycerides

    b. Steroids

    c. Protein

    d. Bile

52. Which of the following vitamins is also known as cyanocobalamin?

    a. A

    b. B_{12}

    c. C

    d. K

53. Which of the following statements about NSAIDs is false?

    a. They are used to decrease inflammation after injuries.

    b. They include aspirin, ibuprofen, naproxen, and acetaminophen.

    c. One of their main side effects is gastrointestinal (GI) upset.

    d. They are used to treat fever.

54. Methotrexate can be used to treat rheumatoid arthritis. What other condition is it used for?

    a. Cancer

    b. Pernicious anemia

    c. Cardiac dysrhythmias

    d. Renal failure

55. Promethazine (Phenergan) is a phenothiazine used to treat which of the following?

    a. Dysrhythmias

    b. Hypertension

    c. Inflammation

    d. Motion sickness

56. In addition to treating rheumatoid arthritis, hydroxychloroquine (Plaquenil) is also used for which of the following?

    a. Cancer

    b. Pernicious anemia

    c. Malaria

    d. Renal failure

57. Isoniazid can affect serum calcium by causing hypercalcemia. A patient receiving this drug is being treated for:

    a. Peptic ulcers

    b. Tuberculosis infection

    c. Viral infection

    d. Inflammation

58. Diazepam (Valium) is used as an antianxiety agent in many hospitalized patients. What other condition is it used for?

    a. Muscle spasms

    b. Osteomyelitis

    c. Parkinson's disease

    d. Immune disorders

CASE STUDY APPLICATIONS

59. Your patient is a 74-year-old man who has primary gout and has just started taking allopurinol (Lopurin), 100 mg daily. He is reporting symptoms of gastric upset and intermittent episodes of extreme pain in the joints.

    a. What education should the nurse provide regarding these symptoms and their treatment?

    b. What education should the nurse provide regarding possible adverse effects?

    c. What laboratory tests should the nurse monitor to determine the longer-term effects of allopurinol?

60. Ms. S is a 28-year-old with type 1 diabetes with renal failure on hemodialysis. You bring her morning medications, which include Rocaltrol and calcium tablets.

    a. She asks you why she is receiving vitamin D and calcium because she does not have a bone disease and is too young for osteoporosis. How do you explain this to her?

    b. What patient teaching regarding vitamin D therapy would you give Ms. S?

    c. What information regarding calcium supplements should you give her?

61. Mrs. R is 78 years old and has been admitted to the hospital with a vertebral compression fracture. Now that her pain has been controlled, she is asking you questions about the prevention of further problems of this nature.

    a. Mrs. R wants to know what causes the bones to become brittle in elderly people. What explanation will you give her?

    b. What drug therapy is likely to be prescribed to treat Mrs. R's osteoporosis?

    c. What education will Mrs. R need regarding the use of her prescriptions for Fosamax and Evista?

CHAPTER 34

DRUGS FOR SKIN DISORDERS

LEARNING OUTCOMES

To view the objectives, please refer to the textbook or MyNursingKit™ at www.mynursingkit.com.

TRUE/FALSE

For Questions 1–9, choose T for true or F for false.

T   F   1. All skin disorders are caused by stresses in the environment.

T   F   2. Pediculicides are pharmacologic agents that kill mites; scabicides kill lice.

T   F   3. An important component of therapy for lice involves removing nits.

T   F   4. The predominant form of drug therapy for sunburn and minor irritation is the application of local anesthetics.

T   F   5. Most acne drugs act by slowing down the turnover of skin cells, especially those surrounding pore openings.

T   F   6. The principal action of isotretinoin (Accutane) is the regulation of skin growth and turnover.

T   F   7. Adverse effects of retinol (vitamin A) are relatively minor and should not be a problem for the patient who is pregnant.

T   F   8. Topical glucocorticoids are the most effective treatment for symptoms of dermatitis.

T   F   9. Numerous drugs are employed to soothe the patient with psoriasis, including emollients, topical glucocorticoids, and immunosuppressant medications.

FILL IN THE BLANK

From the text, find the correct word(s) to complete the statement(s).

10. Drugs used to promote the shedding of old skin are called _____ agents.

11. Mites cause a skin disorder called _____.

12. Vitamin A–like compounds providing resistance to bacterial infection by reducing oil production and the occurrence of clogged pores are called _____.

13. Drugs used to soothe and soften the skin, as in the case of psoriasis, are called _____.

14. Itching associated with dry, scaly skin is called _____.

15. Other than keratolytic agents, two classes of drugs, and _____, offer some protection against acne.

16. A skin disorder with symptoms resembling an allergic reaction is called atopic dermatitis or _____.

17. Small, inflammatory bumps without pus are called _____.

MATCHING

For Questions 18–24, match the drug in Column I with its classification in Column II.

Column I	**Column II**
18. _____ Benzoyl peroxide (BenzaClin)	a. Scabicide/pediculicide
19. _____ Fluticasone (Flonase)	b. Sunburn/minor irritation agent
20. _____ Etretinate (Tegison)	c. Acne and acne-related agent
21. _____ Azelaic acid (Azelex)	d. Topical glucocorticoid
22. _____ Permethrin (Nix)	e. Psoriatic agent
23. _____ Benzocaine (Solarcaine)	
24. _____ Sulfacetamide sodium (AK-Sulf)	

For Questions 25–29, match the symptom in Column I with its description in Column II.

Column I	**Column II**
25. _____ Erythema	a. Blackheads
26. _____ Pruritus	b. Whiteheads
27. _____ Sunburn	c. Intense itching
28. _____ Open comedones	d. Redness
29. _____ Closed comedones	e. "First-degree" injury

MULTIPLE CHOICE

30. Drugs to treat oily skin would most likely be used for which of the following disorders?

    a. Atopic dermatitis

    b. Contact dermatitis

    c. Seborrheic dermatitis

    d. Stasis dermatitis

31. Which of the following medications is also used for the treatment of wrinkles?

    a. Benzoyl peroxide (BenzaClin)

    b. Tretinoin (Retin-A)

    c. Calcipotriene (Dovonex)

    d. Hydroxyurea (Hydrea)

32. Which of the following medications is administered topically for psoriasis?

    a. Calcipotriene (Dovonex)

    b. Acitretin (Soriatane)

    c. Etretinate (Tegison)

    d. Methotrexate (Amethopterin, Folex, Rheumatrex)

33. Which of the following medications would NOT be useful for minor insect bites?

    a. Benzocaine (Solarcaine)

    b. Dibucaine (Nupercainal)

    c. Tetracaine (Pontocaine)

    d. Isotretinoin (Accutane)

34. Which of the following treatments would NOT be used to promote the shedding of old skin?

    a. Resorcinol

    b. Salicylic acid

    c. Sulfur

    d. Benzoyl peroxide

35. Which of the following statements about benzocaine is true?

    a. When applied to the ear, mouth, or throat, it produces minor irritation.

    b. It is more appropriate for sunburn than for pruritus or insect bites.

    c. Drug sensitivity is rare.

    d. It should not be applied to an open wound.

36. Which of the following is an over-the-counter (OTC) medication for acne?

    a. Adapalene (Differin)

    b. Azelaic acid (Azelex)

    c. Benzoyl peroxide (BenzaClin)

    d. Sulfacetamide (Klaron)

37. Exposure to perfume, cosmetics, detergents, or latex is associated with which of the following disorders?

    a. Atopic dermatitis

    b. Contact dermatitis

    c. Seborrheic dermatitis

    d. Stasis dermatitis

38. Topical glucocorticoids are a common treatment for all of the following EXCEPT:

    a. Psoriasis

    b. Rosacea

    c. Pruritus

    d. Dermatitis

39. Which of the following is contraindicated in conjunction with phototherapy for the treatment of psoriasis?

    a. Tar and anthralin

    b. Keratolytic pastes

    c. Psoralens

    d. Cyclosporine

40. Scabicides and pediculicides are contraindicated in all of the following patients EXCEPT:

    a. Children ages 2–10

    b. Children less than 2 years old

    c. Children with seizures

    d. Children who have abrasions, rash, or dermatitis

41. Use of retinoid compounds are contraindicated in patients with all of the following conditions EXCEPT:

    a. Rosacea

    b. Severe depression and suicidal tendencies

    c. Seizures treated with carbamazepine

    d. Diabetes treated with oral agents

42. Which vitamin is synthesized by the skin?

    a. A

    b. D

    c. E

    d. K

DO YOU REMEMBER?

43. Methotrexate may be used to treat psoriasis. Which other condition is it used for?

    a. Gout and rheumatoid arthritis

    b. Rheumatoid arthritis and certain cancers

    c. Systemic fungal infections and certain cancers

    d. Urinary tract infections and peptic ulcers

44. Topical metronidazole (Flagyl) is used to treat rosacea. For which of the following options is it used when given PO or IV?

    a. Crohn's disease

    b. To decrease lipid levels in the blood

    c. Anti-infective therapy

    d. Dysrhythmias

45. What drug is used as a local anesthetic and an antidysrhythmic?

    a. Warfarin (Coumadin)

    b. Propranolol (Inderal)

    c. Infliximab (Remicade)

    d. Lidocaine (Xylocaine)

46. Which of the following is among the first-choice drugs used for allergic rhinitis?

    a. Nonsteroidal anti-inflammatory drugs (NSAIDs)

    b. Sympathomimetics

    c. Glucocorticoids

    d. Cytokines

CASE STUDY APPLICATIONS

47. Ms. G is a 9-year-old brought to the pediatrician by her mother for an immunization. As you give the injection, you notice that the child has nits clinging to her hair. A quick assessment tells you that the child appears to be clean and well cared for. When you point out the problem to her mother, she confesses that she has used an OTC treatment for the lice, which her daughter got at a friend's sleepover. She is obviously uncomfortable and blurts out, "We're not like that—we are clean people." A prescription for Kwell is given to the mother.

    a. What teaching must you do regarding the use of lindane?

    b. Whom must the mother notify of her daughter's pediculosis?

    c. What information can you give the mother and daughter to prevent this problem from recurring?

48. You are working at a walk-in clinic in Florida. A 20-year-old college student visiting from Minnesota on spring break presents with complaints of severe sunburn.

    a. What other assessments would you need?

    b. What interventions might help the pain and other symptoms of sunburn?

    c. Promotion of wellness is one goal in your care plan. What information should be given to the patient regarding prevention and sequelae of sunburn?

49. Zack, a 17-year-old, stops by the school nurse's office to "hang out." After some preliminary conversation, he confides to you that he is worried about his complexion and that nothing he has tried has cleared up his severe acne. He is afraid that he will be "scarred for life" and asks if there are any other medications to help him. He also wants to know why he has such a bad case of acne, and his friend has hardly any.

    a. What can you tell Zack about the causes of acne?

    b. What assessments must be made prior to starting Accutane?

    c. What other information should be assessed regarding Zack's lifestyle and hygiene habits?

CHAPTER 35

DRUGS FOR EYE AND EAR DISORDERS

LEARNING OUTCOMES

To view the objectives, please refer to the textbook or MyNursingKit™ at www.mynursingkit.com.

TRUE/FALSE

For Questions 1–7, choose T for true or F for false.

T   F   1. Drugs that increase the outflow of aqueous humor include miotics, sympathomimetics, prostaglandins, and prostamides.

T   F   2. Sympathomimetics are drugs that cause constriction of the pupils.

T   F   3. One concern with cycloplegic drugs is that they may gain access into the general circulation, causing salivation, tightening of the airways, and other parasympathetic effects.

T   F   4. Of all antiglaucoma agents, beta blockers are used most often to increase the outflow of aqueous humor.

T   F   5. Osmotic diuretics reduce plasma volume and, therefore, represent one approach to reduce the formation of aqueous humor in patients with glaucoma.

T   F   6. In order to provide relief for a range of otic symptoms, glucocorticoids are often used in combination with antibiotics and other drugs.

T   F   7. Earwax buildup is commonly treated in elderly patients.

FILL IN THE BLANK

From the text, find the correct word(s) to complete the statement(s).

8. In patients who have glaucoma, increased intraocular pressure is most often caused by a(n) _____ in the _____ of aqueous humor.

9. A type of slower-developing glaucoma, in which the iris does not cover the trabecular meshwork, is referred to as _____.

10. Drugs that cause the pupils to constrict are called _____.

11. Drugs that cause the pupils to dilate are referred to as _____.

12. Drugs that cause the relaxation of ciliary muscles are called _____.

13. Swimmer's ear is sometimes referred to as _____.

14. Inflammation of the middle ear is called _____.

15. Inflammation of the mastoid sinus is called _____.

16. Another word for earwax is _____.

MATCHING

For Questions 17–22, match the drug in Column I with its action in Column II.

Column I	Column II
17. _____ Pilocarpine HCl (Adsorbocarpine)	a. Increase the outflow of aqueous humor
18. _____ Timolol (Timoptic)	b. Decrease the formation of aqueous humor
19. _____ Acetazolamide (Diamox)	
20. _____ Mannitol (Osmitrol)	
21. _____ Epinephrine borate (Epinal)	
22. _____ Latanoprost (Xalatan)	

For Questions 23–30, match the antiglaucoma drug in Column I with its classification in Column II.

Column I	Column II
23. _____ Pilocarpine (Adsorbocarpine)	a. Miotic, direct-acting cholinergic agent
24. _____ Dorzolamide HCl (Trusopt)	b. Miotic, cholinesterase inhibitor
25. _____ Isosorbide (Ismotic)	c. Sympathomimetic
26. _____ Epinephrine borate (Epinal)	d. Prostaglandin or prostamide
27. _____ Demecarium bromide (Humorsol)	e. Beta blocker
28. _____ Travaprost (Travatan)	f. Direct acting alpha$_2$-adrenergic agent
29. _____ Betaxolol (Betoptic)	g. Carbonic anhydrase inhibitor
30. _____ Apraclonidine (Iopidine)	h. Osmotic diuretic

MULTIPLE CHOICE

31. Which of the following types of medications may contribute to the development of glaucoma?

    a. Beta blockers

    b. Glucocorticoids

    c. Antibiotics

    d. Calcium channel blockers

32. Which of the following best describes closed-angle glaucoma?

    a. Is referred to as chronic, simple glaucoma

    b. Develops when the iris is pushed over the area where the aqueous fluid normally drains

    c. Develops more slowly than open-angle glaucoma

    d. Is best treated by drugs that decrease the formation of aqueous humor

33. Which of the following classes of drugs for eye procedures should NOT be used for patients with glaucoma?

    a. Mydriatic (sympathomimetic) drugs

    b. Cycloplegic (anticholinergic) drugs

    c. Osmotic diuretics

    d. Carbonic anhydrase inhibitors

34. When used for glaucoma, one drawback of prostaglandins is that they:

    a. Change the pigmentation of the eye

    b. Reduce blood pressure

    c. Increase urine output

    d. Block sympathetic impulses

35. Which of the following medications is converted to epinephrine in the eye?

    a. Unoprostone isopropyl (Rescula)

    b. Physostigmine sulfate (Eserine Sulfate)

    c. Dipivefrin hydrochloride (Propine)

    d. Echothiophate iodide (Phospholine Iodide)

36. Which class of drugs used for eye examinations has the potential to produce unfavorable central nervous system (CNS) effects?

    a. Osmotic diuretics

    b. Sympathomimetic drugs

    c. Anticholinergic drugs

    d. Cholinergic agents

37. Major risk factors associated with glaucoma include all of the following EXCEPT:

    a. Hypertension

    b. Migraine headaches

    c. Ethnic origin

    d. Epilepsy

38. Which of the following statements regarding closed-angle (acute) glaucoma is false?

    a. It is usually unilateral.

    b. The iris is pushed over the area where the fluid normally drains.

    c. It is frequently seen in Caucasian persons.

    d. It constitutes an emergency situation.

39. Which of the following statements regarding beta-blocking agents is false?

    a. They are contraindicated in persons who are allergic to sulfa.

    b. They are the most frequently used antiglaucoma drugs.

    c. The mechanism by which they work is not fully understood.

    d. They may produce systemic side effects, such as bronchoconstriction, bradycardia, and hypotension.

40. In which of the following patients would the use of Diamox, a carbonic anhydrase inhibitor, be contraindicated?

    a. A patient with asthma-producing bronchospasms

    b. A patient with an allergy to sulfonamides

    c. A patient with open-angle glaucoma

    d. A patient with a history of third-degree atrioventricular (AV) block

41. You are teaching an elderly patient to instill her own eyedrops. How will you explain the procedure?

    a. Tilt the head back and toward the side of the affected eye.

    b. Tilt the head back and toward the side of the unaffected eye.

    c. Instill the drops to the center of the cornea, blink, and wipe the eye.

    d. Lift the upper lid by the lashes and drop the medication into the sac.

42. When teaching a family member to instill eyedrops for an elderly patient, all of the following should be included EXCEPT:

    a. Apply gentle pressure for 30 seconds to the inner canthus after instilling.

    b. Wait 5 minutes before instilling another type of drops.

    c. There is no need to remove the patient's contact lenses.

    d. Eye medication should be refrigerated.

43. What is the basic course of treatment for ear infection?

    a. Antibiotics

    b. Corticosteroids

    c. Earwax removal agents

    d. Irrigation with a bulb syringe

44. Which of the following regarding chloramphenicol (Chloromycetin Otic) eardrops is false?

    a. It is used primarily in cases of a ruptured eardrum.

    b. It is indicated if the patient has hypersensitivity to the drug.

    c. It is the most commonly used topical antibiotic.

    d. Side effects include burning, redness, rash, and swelling.

45. When instilling eardrops, all of the following are correct EXCEPT:

    a. Run warm water over the bottle to warm the drops.

    b. In an adult patient, the pinna should be held up and back.

    c. The patient should lie on the side opposite the affected ear for 5 minutes after instillation.

    d. The area should not be massaged to prevent systemic drug effects.

DO YOU REMEMBER?

46. Cholinergic agents exert an effect in the body through which type of receptor?

    a. Histaminergic

    b. Muscarinic

    c. Dopaminergic

    d. Serotonergic

47. Beta blockers are examples of which class of antidysrhythmic drugs?

    a. Class I

    b. Class II

    c. Class III

    d. Class IV

48. What is one important respiratory effect of beta blockers?

    a. Bronchospasm

    b. Bronchodilation

    c. Increased release of surfactant

    d. Hyperventilation

49. What is the most serious adverse effect of taking potassium-sparing diuretics and salt substitutes at the same time?

    a. Hyperkalemia

    b. Hypokalemia

    c. Edema

    d. Dehydration

50. In addition to glaucoma, the carbonic anhydrase inhibitor acetazolamide (Diamox) is also prescribed for which of the following?

    a. Seizures

    b. Coagulation disorders

    c. Psoriasis

    d. Malaria

CASE STUDY APPLICATIONS

51. The patient has acute glaucoma. Pilocarpine HCl (Isopto Carpine) has been ordered, 1 drop every 5 minutes for 6 doses. Should the nurse question this order? Why or why not?

52. Mr. M was recently diagnosed with open-angle glaucoma. Intraocular pressure is currently being controlled with miotic medications, including latanoprost (Xalatan). Mr. M wants to know if there is a permanent cure and if continued treatment will be necessary.

    a. Your care plan includes interventions related to patient education. What patient teaching must you do for Mr. M regarding his disease?

    b. One of Mr. M's nursing diagnoses is "Knowledge deficit related to therapeutic regimen as evidenced by patient's inability to tell indications and side effects of antiglaucoma medications." What specific information regarding the use of latanoprost must you as the nurse give Mr. M?

    c. List some general nursing interventions that would be important for a patient with glaucoma.

    d. How would you evaluate the effectiveness of Mr. M's glaucoma medications?

53. Five-year-old Timmy B is brought to the pediatrician's office by his mother, who states that he has been crying, running a temperature of 102, and complaining of an earache. Your assessment reveals bulging, reddened eardrums, and bloody drainage in the left ear. The mother states that she has been using chewable baby aspirin for his fever and that she has another child at home using "eardrops, and he hates those cold things going into his ears." A diagnosis of otitis media is made by the doctor, and an oral antibiotic is prescribed.

    a. What other assessments must you make regarding the use of antibiotics by this patient?

    b. Mrs. B obviously has a lack of knowledge about Timmy's medications and treatments. What interventions could you include in your care plan to address this patient problem?

54. Mrs. I has come to the clinic with complaints of mild hearing loss and a sensation of fullness, with intermittent ringing of the ears. On assessment with the otoscope, you observe a dark mass in the ear canal.

    a. What other assessments should be made prior to treating this problem?

    b. How would the problem be treated?

ANSWER KEY

Chapter 1

1. F   2. F   3. T   4. T   5. F   6. F
7. T   8. T
9. drugs
10. natural alternative
11. therapeutics; pharmaceutics
12. *U.S. Pharmacopeia*, *National Formulary*, American Pharmaceutical Association (APhA)
13. Food, Drug, and Cosmetic
14. clinical phase trials
15. Health Canada
16. Notice of Compliance (NOC); Drug Identification Number (DIN)
17. d   18. c   19. a   20. b   21. f, c, d, e, a, b
22. d   23. c   24. c   25. b   26. d   27. b
28. a   29. d   30. a   31. c   32. c
33. a. Natural alternative therapies usually cost less, especially if patients are choosy about where they obtain these products. In many cases, they can be safer and at least equally or more effective than OTC medications. Also, because natural alternative therapies are naturally produced, they tend to produce relatively fewer side effects, which is definitely an advantage.

    b. Mild constipation is a good example of a situation in which patients might consider changing their diet, eating foods with a higher fiber or bran content. If this does not help, it is not likely that OTC medication will be more helpful. In this case, if symptoms persist, patients should see their health care practitioner, so that prescription drugs can be considered as a part of a more extensive medical therapy.

34. a. It is important to understand that a patient's experience of an unfavorable medication reaction does not necessarily mean that something is wrong with his or her medication. Having an understanding of the drug approval process, however, makes it easier to understand that at least the potential harmful effects of a medication within the general population have been studied. On the other hand, consistent harmful effects have been reported for some products after drugs have reached the market; it is wise to consider this whenever patients make a complaint. Therefore, you should explain that there are many reasons for an unfavorable drug reaction, including expected side effects, drug dose and frequency considerations, the patient's medical history, and other drugs taken concurrently. These and other factors, including the patient's age, body mass, and genetic variables, must also be considered. In all cases, if a medication appears to be harmful, patients should immediately discontinue taking their medication and consult with their health care practitioner.

    b. Unfavorable reactions to prescription medications should be reported immediately to the health care practitioner and/or pharmacist, whereas unfavorable reactions to OTC medications should be reported directly to the pharmacist or appropriate representatives from the FDA (Health Canada for Canadian citizens), depending on where and how the patient obtained the drug. Problems with natural alternative therapies might also be reported to the FDA or Health Canada.

35. a. Because Mrs. M has not been exposed to anthrax, antibiotic use is not recommended. The antibiotic is expensive, can cause significant side effects, and, most importantly, can promote the development of bacterial strains that are resistant to antibiotics.

    b. Anthrax vaccine is available. It takes 18 months to complete the six injections. At this point, the CDC recommends vaccination for laboratory personnel only who work with anthrax, military personnel in high-risk areas, and those who deal with animal products imported from areas where the disease is endemic.

Chapter 2

1. F   2. F   3. T   4. T   5. F   6. F
7. T
8. therapeutic
9. pharmacologic
10. mechanism of action
11. chemical
12. combination drugs
13. addiction
14. scheduled
15. restricted
16. d   17. c   18. b   19. e   20. a   21. a
22. e   23. c   24. b   25. d   26. c   27. c

28. a   29. c   30. c   31. a   32. b   33. a
34. a   35. a

36. a. Penicillin V is a category B drug; therefore, it should be OK to take this medication.

    b. Acetaminophen is a category B drug; therefore, it should be OK to take this medication.

    c. Naproxen is a category B drug; therefore, it should be OK to take this medication.

    d. Castor oil is a category X drug and should NOT be taken during pregnancy.

    e. Diazepam is a category D drug and should NOT be taken during pregnancy. Diazepam is a Schedule IV drug.

37. a. Generic and trade products have identical doses; however, the ingredients in the generic product may be slightly different. In many states, the pharmacist is allowed to dispense generic equivalents unless the patient or nurse specifies that a trade product is required. In Florida, if a drug is on the negative drug formulary list, it must be dispensed in its trade form only. As a nurse, it is best to check the state requirements for dispensing of trade versus generic products.

    b. Tylenol is an analgesic nonnarcotic. It is not a controlled substance. In the United States, controlled substances are drugs whose use is restricted by the Controlled Substances Act of 1970.

Chapter 3

1. F   2. F   3. T   4. F   5. F   6. F
7. T   8. T
9. enteral
10. topical
11. pharmacokinetic
12. Viscosity; solubility
13. oral
14. Sublingual
15. Suppositories; enemas
16. intravenous
17. intramuscular
18. intrathecal; epidural
19. transdermal
20. Transmucosal

21. c   22. b   23. b   24. a   25. c   26. b
27. c   28. a   29. b   30. b   31. b   32. c
33. a   34. a   35. b   36. b   37. c   38. a
39. b   40. a   41. c   42. b   43. d   44. d
45. c   46. d   47. a   48. b   49. b   50. b
51. c   52. d   53. b   54. d   55. c

56. a. The nurse should take a detailed personal, family, and sexual health history when assisting the patient in a choice of contraception.

    b. Oral contraceptive agents are effective and convenient; however, missing a daily dose means risking pregnancy. Therefore, for an active lifestyle, this may not be the most desirable approach. On the other hand, an oral medication may be less bothersome than injections, patches, or vaginal inserts. Injections or implants may last a long time, but they may be initially painful or subject to infection. In addition, these approaches may be uncomfortable, as may vaginal inserts. Vaginal inserts might be used less routinely because they are sometimes messy, inconvenient, and less reliable. The nurse should help the patient weigh every disadvantage against the convenience of taking medication less frequently.

57. a. Because the patient is nauseous and has diarrhea, oral medications or suppositories would probably not be recommended unless the nausea and diarrhea were not severe enough to interfere with the drug therapy. Because the source of discomfort is the gastrointestinal tract, topical drugs would most likely do little good to relieve discomfort; in elderly patients, the skin is usually sensitive. Alternatives might be drugs administered by the parenteral route—for example, in an intramuscular or subcutaneous injection.

    b. Effectiveness of the route of medication can be evaluated by collecting data about the resolution of presenting symptoms.

Chapter 4

1. F   2. T   3. F   4. T   5. T   6. F
7. T   8. T   9. F   10. F
11. absorption; distribution; metabolism; excretion
12. blood-brain; blood-placental; blood-testicular
13. Metabolism
14. Prodrugs
15. first-pass effect
16. metabolites
17. enterohepatic recirculation
18. half-life
19. Pharmacodynamics
20. receptor
21. Potency; efficacy

22. b   23. a   24. b   25. a   26. a   27. a
28. a   29. b   30. b   31. a   32. a   33. b
34. b   35. b   36. a   37. b   38. c   39. b
40. d   41. c   42. c   43. d   44. d   45. a
46. c   47. a   48. d   49. a   50. b

51. a. Because Mr. P is moderately obese, the medications may be dissolved in the fat and accumulate there and then slowly be released. Hypertension and diabetes can alter drug distribution,

because these disorders are associated with compromised renal function. When renal function is compromised, drug dosing must be reduced to account for changes in metabolic and excretion function.

b. Mr. P's anxiety should be reduced. Half-life of the drug should be considered by the nurse. If the patient is experiencing side effects of the antianxiety drugs, then the nurse should consider renal and hepatic function as a potential problem, increasing the plasma half-life.

c. The primary site of excretion for all medications is the kidney. The nurse should be checking intake and output on this patient.

52. a. Mr. A has been abusing alcohol, which will affect hepatic function. He is 60 years old and, therefore, has some degree of vessel narrowing.

b. Because of the history of alcohol abuse and the age of the patient, medication dosing may be reduced to lessen the chance of toxicity.

c. The nurse should assess the renal system. If renal blood flow has been impaired, then excretion of medications will be slow and side or toxic effects may be seen in the postprocedure period.

53. a. Determine the age of the patient. Identify how often the analgesic is used for pain relief and how effective the medication has been. Identify if the dosage is standard and safe. Evaluate the therapeutic index for this drug.

b. Chronic pain related to history of migraine headaches

c. Has there been enough time for the medication to be absorbed and distributed? Does the patient need a more potent drug? Is the formulation of this drug not appropriate for this patient? Are drug-drug interactions occurring? Are drug-food interactions occurring?

54. a. What antibiotics are the patients taking? Are the doses standard, safe, and potent? Have the patients taken the drugs long enough to consider the slow results unreasonable? Is this an effectiveness issue?

b. The patient exhibits the following signs of wound healing: well-approximated wound edges, no drainage 48 hours after the wound is closed, no inflammatory response past day 5 after the injury.

c. Wound edges opening, drainage, inflammation, pain, fever

Chapter 5

1. F   2. F   3. F   4. T   5. T
6. Subjective
7. etiologies
8. active participants
9. nursing process

10. nursing diagnosis
11. nonadherence or noncompliance
12. f   13. e   14. d   15. c   16. g   17. b
18. a   19. c   20. d   21. b   22. a   23. b
24. a   25. d   26. b   27. c   28. a   29. c
30. a   31. b   32. b   33. c   34. a
35. Potential nursing diagnosis includes:

a. Risk for Injury, related to improper use of drug therapy and elevated glucose levels

b. Noncompliance to treatment related to a failure to follow treatment plan.

Goal 1: Patient will adhere to medication regimen.

Goal 2: Patient will initiate diet and exercise changes and participate in treatment plan.

36. Barriers to expect include language, culture, lifestyle, education, low-income, and healthcare beliefs. A priority intervention is to establish the need for, and use of, an interpreter to communicate with the patient. This will enable the nurse to obtain an accurate assessment and be able to communicate a plan of care to the patient. It also reduces the chances for legal implications.

37. The potential exists for withdrawal symptom (related to the substance abuse) which may require additional medication for pain relief. Also, there is a potential for noncompliance to treatment related to drug dependency.

Goal 1: Patient will follow established plan of care both as an inpatient and outpatient.

Goal 2: Patient will enroll in a substance abuse recovery program and be in compliance with goals of the program.

The desired outcome will be for a complete recovery from the trauma and substance abuse.

Chapter 6

1. F   2. F   3. F   4. T
5. Dietary Supplement Health and Education
6. reduce; medications
7. anticoagulants
8. d   9. b   10. a   11. c   12. e   13. c
14. a   15. d   16. d   17. c   18. c   19. b
20. a   21. d   22. d   23. a
24. a. Modern medical research often employs animal models that may not respond the same way as humans. The herb may have active ingredients in a specific region and may interact with local foods. Mr. K must also realize that the herb may have slowed his memory disorder but perhaps not as dramatically as he expected. No herb or prescription medicine is effective enough to delay or prevent all diseases.

b. Herbs may contain dozens of active chemicals, many of which have not yet been isolated, studied, or even identified. It is possible that many of these substances work together synergistically and may not have the same activity if isolated. Scientists may not be studying the right combination of factors for a long enough time to demonstrate an effect.

25. a. The patient may be experiencing serotonin syndrome caused by the combination of the Prozac and the St. John's wort.

b. Combining St. John's wort with tricyclic antidepressants, such as Elavil or Tofranil, may cause serotonin syndrome. MAOIs in combination with St. John's wort may cause hypertensive crisis.

Chapter 7

1. F   2. T   3. T   4. F   5. F   6. T
7. F   8. T   9. T   10. F
11. alcohol; nicotine
12. opium; marijuana; cocaine
13. dose; length of therapy
14. physical dependence; psychological dependence
15. Addiction
16. crack cocaine
17. benzodiazepine
18. methadone
19. tolerance
20. I
21. Nicotine
22. withdrawal
23. a   24. c   25. c   26. d   27. b   28. b
29. d   30. a   31. c   32. a   33. a   34. b
35. a   36. a   37. b   38. a   39. b   40. b
41. c   42. a   43. d   44. d   45. c   46. d
47. a   48. d   49. b
50. a. Marijuana can cause lung damage and the chance for cancer of the lung.

b. Marijuana causes psychological dependence. It is also considered the "gateway" drug: It opens the patient to opportunities for poor judgment and the possibility of taking other drugs when the person is "high" on marijuana.

c. Lung cancer is a risk in those people who smoke marijuana.

51. a. There is substantial evidence to suggest that genetics plays a major role in addiction. However, many factors could increase the likelihood of someone abusing alcohol as well as other addictive drugs. If a person has a genetic predisposition to substance abuse, it is best to weigh the risks of addiction carefully before consuming alcohol or other addicting substances.

b. When did the patient last consume alcohol? How much alcohol is usually consumed in a day/week? Has the patient ever had withdrawal symptoms? Has the patient ever been to an alcohol treatment program? What is the patient's current mental status? What is the patient's nutritional status? What is the patient's skin integrity like?

c. One nursing diagnosis is chronic low self-esteem related to substance abuse. The patient outcome is stable self-esteem. A second nursing diagnosis is compromised family coping related to substance abuse. The patient outcome is that the family will understand the behaviors needed to support a drug-free family environment and cope with the recovery process. A third nursing diagnosis is risk for violence related to altered perceptions and poor impulse control. The patient outcome is no violence experienced; altered perceptions are prevented or treated early. A final nursing diagnosis is deficient knowledge related to lack of understanding of the use and abuse of alcohol. The patient outcome is that the patient will express the causes and treatment of addictions and will be able to express the prevention behaviors necessary to be drug free.

Chapter 8

1. F   2. T   3. F   4. F   5. T   6. T
7. b   8. b   9. a   10. a
11. central; peripheral
12. autonomic
13. fight-or-flight; rest-and-digest
14. presynaptic; synapse cleft; postsynaptic
15. Norepinephrine; acetylcholine
16. adrenergics; cholinergic
17. parasympathetic; sympathetic
18. Adrenergic
19. adrenergic (or sympathetic)
20. Cholinergic
21. e   22. b   23. c   24. d   25. a   26. c
27. b   28. a   29. e   30. d   31. b   32. c
33. a   34. d   35. c   36. d   37. d   38. a
39. d   40. a   41. a   42. c   43. a   44. b
45. b   46. a   47. b   48. c   49. c   50. a
51. c   52. a   53. a   54. d   55. c

56.

Drug	Class	Effect or Action	Interactions	
Benadryl	Anticholinergic	Dries secretions, causing difficulty for patients with COPD	Increases heart rate and blood pressure	Causes drowsiness, urinary hesitancy, and retention
Propranolol	Adrenergic blocker	Decreases bronchodilation, causing difficulty for patients with COPD	Decreases heart rate and blood pressure, causes orthostatic hypotension	Causes drowsiness and possible depression
Prazosin	Adrenergic blocker	Decreases bronchodilation, causing difficulty for patients with COPD	Vasodilation to decrease blood pressure, allows increased heart rate	Causes urinary hesitancy
Proventil	Adrenergic	Causes bronchodilation	Increases blood pressure and heart rate	

These actions work against each other in the cardiovascular areas and respiratory areas.

a. Potential nursing diagnoses would include:
1. Ineffective airway clearance due to drying of secretions caused by Benadryl and interference with bronchodilation when propranolol is given
2. Possible altered urinary elimination: retention or hesitancy related to use of prazosin and Benadryl
3. Possible altered cardiac output: decrease related to use of prazosin, propranolol

b. Nursing interventions that can be done to decrease possible problems or interactions include:
1. Identify interactions and review with the physician when appropriate.
2. Increase hydration to 3 L/day to decrease risk of drying of secretions, causing altered airway clearance.
3. Monitor for signs of orthostatic hypotension and possible decreases or increases in blood pressure or pulse.
4. Monitor intake and output to be sure the patient maintains urine output and experiences no urinary dysfunction due to adverse medication effects.

57. a. To identify a nursing diagnosis, the nurse would assess the following:
Muscle strength
Knowledge of the medication regime
Compliance with medication regime
Unusual activities of daily living
Unusual medical conditions
Previous medications and present medications
Administration of medications

b. Nursing diagnoses would include the following:
Risk for injury
Impaired physical mobility
Knowledge deficit

c. Nursing interventions could include the following:

Impaired physical mobility: Assess for muscle strength and neurologic status.

Risk for injury: Assist with mobility; monitor for proper use of mobility equipment: canes, walkers, and transfers; monitor for safety hazards in the home; monitor for ability to chew and swallow.

Knowledge deficit: Monitor for the patient's knowledge before and after teaching about medications and safety teaching.

Chapter 9

1. T   2. F   3. T   4. T   5. F   6. T
7. F   8. F
9. generalized anxiety
10. limbic; reticular activating
11. Anxiolytics; hypnotics
12. GABA receptor-chloride

13. benzodiazepines
14. Barbiturates
15. Respiratory depression
16. IV; II
17. Seasonal affective disorder
18. sedative and sedative-hypnotic

19. b	20. a	21. c	22. c	23. d	24. d
25. a	26. e	27. a	28. c	29. b	30. b
31. a	32. a	33. d	34. c	35. d	36. c
37. a	38. d	39. b	40. b	41. b	42. c
43. b	44. b	45. b	46. d	47. d	48. a

49. a. Nursing assessments prior to giving Versed include:

> Allergies to benzodiazepines or chemically similar drugs
>
> Liver and renal function
>
> History of any chronic respiratory conditions
>
> History of depression or alcohol or drug abuse
>
> Medications taken routinely and when taken last, including herbals

    b. Nursing interventions would include:

> Resuscitation equipment and airway
>
> Romazicon as benzodiazepine blocker
>
> Ventilator
>
> Someone to take the patient home after the procedure
>
> Monitor vital signs every 5 to 15 minutes, especially the respiratory rate and depth
>
> Monitor the patient's level of consciousness and responsiveness

    c. To evaluate the effectiveness of intervention, the nurse would use the following:

> The patient has no injury related to the administration of Versed.
>
> The patient has normal vital signs during the administration of Versed.

50. a. Sleep pattern disturbance related to anxiety response

    b. Nursing interventions would include:

> Explore potential contributing factors.
>
> Maintain bedtime routine as per patient preference.
>
> Provide comfort measures to induce sleep:
>
> > Nonpharmacologic techniques
> >
> > Back rub
> >
> > Light bedtime snack
> >
> > A regular time to sleep
> >
> > Avoidance of napping during the day
> >
> > Decreased caffeine, chocolate, nicotine, and other stimulant use in the second half of the day
> >
> > Limited alcohol consumption
> >
> > Exercise at least 2–3 hours before bedtime
> >
> > Hot bath 1 hour before sleep
> >
> > Comfortable sleeping environment
> >
> > Stress reduction and relaxation just prior to sleep
> >
> > Relief of pain or discomfort prior to sleep

    c. Pharmacologic techniques will provide information to the patient regarding pharmacotherapeutics. Benzodiazepines would be the drug of first choice for sleep. However, all of these drugs will cause interruption of REM sleep and, therefore, should not be continued for more than 1 week. Certain OTC drugs are normally anticholinergics and again interrupt REM sleep, can cause a hangover, and should not be used for more than 1 week.

Chapter 10

1. T	2. F	3. T	4. F	5. F	6. T
7. T	8. T	9. T			

10. affective
11. major depression; bipolar disorder
12. tricyclic antidepressants (TCA); selective serotonin-reuptake inhibitors (SSRIs); monoamine oxidase inhibitors (MAOIs)
13. SSRIs
14. TCAs
15. lithium
16. attention deficit disorder (ADD)
17. CNS stimulants
18. Seasonal affective
19. mood stabilizers; mania; depression

20. f	21. e	22. d	23. b	24. c	25. a
26. a	27. c	28. b	29. e	30. d	31. d
32. c	33. e	34. b	35. a	36. d	37. c
38. d	39. d	40. d	41. d	42. d	43. c
44. c	45. b	46. d	47. b	48. a	49. c
50. b	51. c	52. c	53. a	54. b	55. a
56. d					

57. a. Risk for injury related to adverse effects of lithium

    b. The nurse should assess for the following:

> **Knowledge of side effects:** dizziness, drowsiness, nausea, metallic taste, tremors, vomiting, and diarrhea
>
> **Laboratory studies:** renal and kidney function, blood levels of lithium
>
> **Interactions:** diuretics and low-sodium diet possibly leading to lithium toxicity
>
> **History:** allergies or previous renal or cardiac conditions
>
> **Mental and emotional status:** previous suicide attempts or present intent
>
> Knowledge of whom to notify in case of adverse or toxic effects of lithium
>
> Knowledge of adverse and toxic effects of lithium

c. The goal is to demonstrate the following:

Understanding of drug effects and precautions

Improvement in mood stability

Ability to notify or seek help when questions or problems arise

No injury related to adverse effects of lithium

58. *Goals for the Patient*   *Evaluation*
    (Patient Will Show or Report)

Goals for the Patient	Evaluation
Improved affect or mood	No longer has suicidal ideation, engages in normal daily activities
Improved sleep patterns	Can sleep through the night, stays asleep, and falls asleep easily
Decreasing episodes of side effects	Has decreased headaches, nausea, drowsiness since beginning medications
Continuation of medication regimen	Continues to take medications as ordered

Chapter 11

1. T   2. F   3. T   4. T   5. F
6. schizophrenia
7. chronic; acute
8. months to years; hours to days
9. positive; negative
10. cause (etiology); brain damage; medication overdose; depression; alcoholism; genetics; drug addiction
11. hallucinations; delusions; disorganized thoughts; disorganized speech patterns
12. interest; motivation; responsiveness; pleasure
13. antipsychotic
14. dopamine (D_2)
15. schizophrenia; extrapyramidal
16. b   17. a   18. a   19. a   20. c   21. a
22. c   23. d   24. b   25. c   26. f   27. b
28. d   29. g   30. a   31. e   32. c   33. h
34. i   35. b   36. c   37. d   38. b   39. d
40. b   41. b   42. c   43. b   44. a   45. a
46. a   47. c   48. a   49. c   50. d   51. c
52. b
53. Need from AU
54. a. Interventions used for the diagnosis of knowledge deficit include:

Assess the patient's readiness to learn based on the emotional response of the patient.

Provide health teaching related to Clozaril:

Can cause drowsiness, dry mouth, hypotension

Does not cause as many problems with EPS as Thorazine does

Get up slowly to prevent dizziness and falls due to orthostatic hypotension.

Avoid activities requiring mental alertness until the effects of the medication are known.

Avoid alcohol and other CNS depressants.

Weekly laboratory testing is required to monitor for agranulocytosis.

Report any evidence of infection: sore throat and mild fever.

Instruct the patient on the best time to take the medication and what to do for missed doses.

b. Evaluation will include the following:

Patient will report to laboratory and physician appointments as requested for laboratory work.

Patient will not experience injury (falls) related to dizziness, sedation, ataxia.

Patient remains compliant with the therapeutic regimen prescribed.

Patient verbalizes understanding of the medical regimen, adverse effects of the medication, and need to be compliant.

55. Assessments include the following:

Vital signs: temperature, pulse, blood pressure, and body weight.

Behavior and appearances: dietary intake, activities of daily living, and socialization with others.

Symptoms of condition: hallucinations, delusions, enjoyment of life, personal hygiene, speech patterns, and motor movement.

Monitor for side effects and adverse effects of medications, such as akathisia, abnormal movements, dizziness, drowsiness, constipation, photosensitivity, or orthostatic hypotension.

Let the patient know that side effects will decrease with time on the medication.

Any past history of seizures; medication can influence the seizure threshold.

Assess plans for pregnancy or if any contraceptives are being used.

Monitor for fluid volume deficit by monitoring I and O and weight daily. Teach the patient to increase oral intake to maintain hydration.

Monitor for improvement in symptoms of the condition. Worsening of the condition should be reported immediately.

Monitor compliance with the medication regimen.

Assess present medications or herbs that may interact with the new medication.

Chapter 12

1. F   2. T   3. T   4. F   5. T   6. T
7. T   8. T   9. T
10. autonomic
11. acetylcholine

12. Alzheimer's disease

13. Alzheimer's disease; multiple strokes

14. acetylcholine

15. genetic

16. antipsychotic; extrapyramidal

17. hypotension; tachycardia; muscle twitching; mood changes

18. cognitive; behavioral; daily activities

19. acetylcholinesterase inhibitors; functioning

20. muscle spasms

21. analgesics; anti-inflammatory agents; antispasmodic

22. spasticity

23. dystonia

24. tetany

25. b	26. a	27. c	28. a	29. b	30. c
31. a	32. a	33. b	34. c	35. i	36. h
37. g	38. e	39. f	40. a	41. c	42. d
43. b	44. a	45. b	46. b	47. a	48. a
49. b	50. a	51. a	52. a	53. d	54. d
55. a	56. c	57. a	58. b	59. a	60. d
61. c	62. c	63. b	64. a	65. b	66. d
67. b	68. c	69. a	70. a	71. b	72. a
73. c	74. b	75. d	76. c	77. d	78. a

79. a. The nursing diagnosis is risk for injury related to drug effects and unresolved symptoms of parkinsonism. This diagnosis relates to sedation as a side effect of anticholinergics and of interactions with other possible CNS depressants, such as Zoloft. The tremors and involuntary movements also cause possible balance problems. Orthostatic hypotension is also a side effect that causes instability of balance.

b. The patient will have no injury related to the side effects of medications or the condition (Parkinson's disease).

80. a. The priority diagnosis at this point would be risk of injury related to possible adverse effects of drugs and interactions.

b. Interventions would include:

Assess for interactions between medications in the regimen:

Tricyclics and benzodiazepines can potentiate their CNS depression, causing sedation and sleep deprivation.

Assess for side effects of the medications:

Sedation, vomiting, diarrhea, obstructed urine flow, insomnia, abnormal dreaming, aggression, syncope, depression, headache, irritability, fatigue, urinary incontinence, and restlessness.

Provide instructions for proper administration:

Give at bedtime and once daily.

Maintain a regular medication schedule.

Provide assistance to the patient when memory is impaired.

Assess for contraindicated conditions or medications:

Hypotension, bradycardia, hyperthyroid, peptic ulcer disease.

Teach safety precautions for side effects of the medications: no hot showers, arise slowly, have something to hold on to during ambulation when needed.

Include the family and patient in the management of the patient's condition.

Collaborate with other departments as needed: PT, OT, home health care.

Assess for caregiver strain.

Monitor for improvement with the patient's short-term memory or behaviors while on medications.

81. a. Limited use of the affected muscle, heat or cold packs, hydrotherapy, ultrasound, exercises, massage, and manipulation may help decrease Ms. H's lower back pain.

b. Ms. H needs to know that dizziness, dry mouth, rash, and a fast pulse rate with palpitations may be noted while using this drug. Another, but rare, reaction is swelling of the tongue. She should not take this drug with alcohol, phenothiazines, or MAO inhibitors due to unfavorable reactions.

c. Ask the patient to rate her pain on a scale of 1 to 10 and see if improvement is noted after using the drug. Monitor muscle tone, ROM, and improved ability to do ADLs. These should increase if the drug is effective.

d. The patient should be instructed in proper body mechanics while lifting, sitting, or engaging in other musculoskeletal movement activities.

82. a. Ms. B needs to know that Botox injections are indicated for moderate to severe frown lines. They are not for crow's feet. She also needs to know that they will, however, smooth the lines between the brows temporarily and must be repeated every 3 to 4 months. Although botulinum toxin is a poison in higher quantities, it is safe for use in tiny injections.

b. Side effects of Botox include headache, nausea, flulike symptoms, temporary blepharoptosis, mild pain, erythema at the site of injection, and muscle weakness.

83. a. Mr. P should have a thorough assessment of his physical condition, especially vital signs, skin condition, mobility or lack of it, neurologic function, self-care ability, and nutritional status. The nurse should also determine the adherence to his medication regimen, side effects, and the outcome the family expects.

b. Physical therapy exercises might decrease the severity of his symptoms. These include stretching to help prevent contractures, muscle group strengthening exercises, and repetitive motion exercises. Surgery for tendon release or to sever the nerve-muscle pathway might be used in an extreme situation.

c. Mr. P and his family should be instructed to report any significant changes in his level of consciousness, such as confusion, hallucinations, lethargy, and decreased speech ability. Also, palpitations, chest pain, dyspnea, visual disturbances, and unusual fatigue should be reported to the doctor. Treatment should not be discontinued abruptly. Taking the medications with food should decrease GI upset. Decreased urinary output, distended abdomen, and discomfort should be reported. Dry mouth may be treated with sips of water, sugarless candy, or gum if the patient is able to use this.

d. The family and patient need to be instructed on gentle ROM and other physical therapy as indicated by the physician. Safety measures include rearranging the home to decrease the risk of falls or accidents and placing needed objects within Mr. P's reach.

Chapter 13

1. T   2. F   3. T   4. T   5. T   6. T
7. T   8. F
9. acute; chronic
10. infection; trauma; metabolic disorders; vascular diseases; neoplastic disorders
11. oral contraceptives
12. folate
13. sleep; strobe; flickering
14. Febrile; 3; 5; fever (or temperature)
15. Tegretol
16. Partial; complete
17. Zarontin
18. Valium (diazepam); Dilantin (phenytoin)
19. Status epilepticus; respirations (or breathing)
20. brain
21. airway
22. seizures
23. abnormal; suppress
24. 3; months
25. f   26. e   27. b   28. a   29. c   30. g
31. d   32. a   33. a   34. b   35. a   36. b
37. c   38. d   39. c   40. b   41. b   42. a
43. d   44. a   45. d   46. d   47. c   48. b
49. a   50. b   51. d   52. c   53. c   54. a
55. a
56. a. Possible risk of injury related to medication administration: Inappropriate administration of Dilantin IV can lead to emboli, hypoventilation, hypotension, venous irritation, seizures, or decreased level of consciousness.

b. Nursing interventions for administration of Dilantin IV:

Use saline only to mix Dilantin.

Infuse no faster than 50 mg/min.

Use an IV line with filter.

Check for infiltration often, because it is a soft tissue irritant.

Use a large vein or central venous catheter only.

Never use Dilantin IM.

Avoid hand veins to prevent local vasoconstriction.

Prime the IV line with saline if hanging piggyback.

Monitor for LOC changes after seizure.

Keep side rails up and padded.

Have emergency equipment available.

Monitor for hypotension or depressed respirations during administration.

57. a. Top priority diagnosis: knowledge deficit related to new medical condition and new medication for management of seizures as evidenced by patient asking questions

b. Interventions include:

Assess what the patient knows about epilepsy, seizures, and management.

Assess for any misunderstandings about the medication and treatment regime.

Provide information to the patient regarding the following:

Medications will be dosed at the lowest dosage to prevent seizures, which will decrease the amount of side effects expected.

The medication dosages will be increased as needed if seizures continue.

Other medications might be added or drugs might be changed as needed to control seizures.

Seizures will be controlled best if the patient is compliant with the medication schedule.

Patient will need to return for laboratory appointments and follow-up physician visit to evaluate the therapeutic effect.

Side effects that might be expected initially include dizziness, ataxia, diplopia, and a change of urine color to pink, red, or brown.

The dizziness and drowsiness will decrease as the medication is continued.

More serious side effects should be reported to the physician.

Drugs to avoid: Many medications interact with phenytoin. The patient must inform the physician that he is on phenytoin before any medications are added. The pharmacist might also be consulted before OTC medications and herbals or supplements are added.

No foods need to be avoided, but supplements of folic acid, calcium, and vitamin D will impair the Dilantin. The nurse should give the patient a list of foods that contain folic acid, calcium, and vitamin D. These foods should not be taken in large quantities, although they do not need to be avoided.

Chapter 14

1. F   2. F   3. T   4. F   5. F   6. T
7. F   8. T   9. T
10. narcotics; nonnarcotics
11. anti-inflammatory; antipyretic
12. unripe seeds of the poppy plant
13. tension
14. aura
15. nociceptor
16. anxiety; depression; fatigue
17. character; nature
18. stop; prevent
19. triptans; ergot alkaloids; serotonin
20. intracranial vessels; orally; parenterally; nasally
21. d   22. c   23. a   24. b   25. e   26. d
27. a   28. e   29. c   30. a   31. e   32. e
33. f   34. d   35. a   36. c   37. b   38. e
39. a   40. c   41. c   42. d   43. b   44. a
45. c   46. d   47. a   48. d   49. a   50. b
51. c   52. c   53. b   54. d   55. b   56. c
57. a   58. c
59. a. Interventions include:
    Assess the psychosocial situation of the patient because anxiety, fatigue, and pain will increase the sensation of pain.
    Analyze the cultural aspects of the patient's pain.
    Assess the knowledge of the patient about addiction and use of narcotic analgesics.
    Teach the patient nonpharmacologic aspects of pain control: relaxation, massage, thermal packs, biofeedback.
    Discuss the source of pain and the therapeutic management of the patient's pain, including using narcotic pain reliever only after less potent medications are attempted first.
    Teach the patient to assess levels of pain with objective methods to quantify pain in order to better evaluate management of pain.
    Teach the patient to journal to identify triggers for the pain.
    b. The outcomes are the patient will report less pain after interventions and more relief from pain management techniques, both pharmacologic and nonpharmacologic.
60. a. Interventions include:
    Assess the medication regimen used by the patient.
    Educate the patient on possible nonpharmacologic approaches: relaxation, biofeedback, massage, thermal therapy.
    Educate the patient on triggers that can cause migraines. Help the patient identify triggers that might apply.

Teach the patient appropriate administration techniques of the medications: Take Percodan as the aura begins and not to wait until the headache is severe.

Teach the patient to evaluate the level of pain and evaluate the improvement using the pain scale of choice.

Encourage the patient to revisit the physician if no improvement has been made with the present medications. Encourage the patient to request or ask if additional medications might be helpful.

b. Goals include the following:

Patient will identify triggers to migraines and eliminate the triggers.

Patient will gain comfort by using nonpharmacologic approaches to migraine discomfort.

Patient will identify a decrease in discomfort after the medication is taken.

Empower the patient to seek medication or measures in addition to those previously named.

Chapter 15

1. F   2. T   3. F   4. F   5. F   6. F
7. surface (or regional)
8. infiltration (or field block)
9. consciousness
10. IV; inhaled
11. pain following surgery
12. sensations; consciousness
13. location; extent of desired anesthesias
14. sensation; motor activity
15. opiates; anxiolytics; barbiturates; neuromuscular blockers
16. balanced; lowered
17. e   18. a   19. b   20. c   21. e   22. b
23. b   24. d,e   25. e   26. d   27. c   28. e
29. e   30. a   31. d   32. e   33. b   34. e
35. c   36. h   37. g   38. f   39. d   40. d
41. a   42. b   43. c   44. d   45. c   46. b
47. c   48. a   49. a   50. d   51. b   52. b
53. d   54. a   55. b   56. b
57. a. The nursing diagnosis is knowledge deficit related to upcoming surgery and unknown medication regime.
    b. Interventions include preoperative surgical preparation and teaching:
    Preoperative medications are given to relieve anxiety and provide sedation.
    Anticholinergics are given to dry secretions to prevent pneumonia and aspiration.
    Pain medications are given to aid in pain control.
    IV medication is given to cause rapid unconsciousness.

After IV medication takes effect, the patient is given an inhaled anesthesia.

Muscle relaxants are given to provide relaxation, during which time the patient will breathe with use of a ventilator.

Postoperative medications will include analgesics for the patient and antiemetics, if needed, to prevent vomiting.

Assess the patient's understanding of the information given.

Ask for patient questions.

58. a. The nursing diagnosis is anxiety related to anticipated pain of invasive procedure as evidenced by inability to concentrate; appearance of nervousness, apprehension, and tension; restlessness; and hyperattentiveness.

b. Assessment data include rapid, pressured speech; tremulousness; restlessness; scanning of room; and asking of questions.

c. Interventions would include:

Assist the patient to reduce the level of anxiety by reassuring and staying with the patient.

Speak slowly and calmly when giving information.

Ask about any physical problems and history as well as present medications.

Give clear, concise information when teaching about the medications to be used.

Discuss alternate methods of relaxation.

Help establish short-term goals and reinforce positive responses to questions and actions.

Initiate health teaching in short, concise statements and move at the patient's rate.

Monitor vital signs and any evidence of shortness of breath or chest pain.

d. Goals for the patient include:

The patient will demonstrate a decrease in anxiety as shown by slower speech patterns, decreased vital signs, and the ability to repeat instruction-and-answer questions in a focused method.

The patient will relate information offered during the teaching session relating to the upcoming procedure.

The patient will relate information that has been taught throughout the teaching session.

e. Vital signs are normal. The patient repeats instructions and answers questions appropriately.

Chapter 16

1. F   2. F   3. T   4. T   5. F   6. F
7. F   8. T   9. F   10. T
11. hyperlipidemia
12. plaque
13. triglycerides; phospholipids; steroids

14. cholesterol; triglycerides; phospholipids
15. statin
16. statins/HMG CoA reductase inhibitors
17. a. bile acid sequestrants
    b. statins
    c. niacin
    d. fibric acid agents
18. b   19. a   20. d   21. c   22. a   23. c
24. b   25. b   26. d   27. c   28. d   29. a
30. b   31. a   32. c   33. c   34. d   35. b
36. b   37. a   38. d   39. d   40. c   41. b
42. c   43. a   44. c   45. c

46. a. Aspirin is an OTC analgesic with anticoagulant action that can relieve pain and prevent stroke. Nifedipine is a calcium channel blocker that is commonly prescribed for hypertension. Likewise, chlorothiazide is an antihypertensive diuretic.

b. Mr. L has a history of heart disease and hypertension with highly elevated lipid levels. Therapy with a statin drug is indicated.

c. Mr. L should reduce his dietary intake of lipids and expand his exercise program.

47. a. When medications fail to work, the nurse should ascertain whether or not the patient is taking the drugs as prescribed. Given that Ms. H is taking her medication, she may have changed her dietary habits to include more lipids. Some patients mistakenly believe that the drug alone will lower their lipid levels and that dietary restrictions are unnecessary.

b. The physician may choose to raise the dose of Lipitor to 80 mg/day and wait 6 to 8 weeks to determine if the increased dose is effective. An alternative choice is to add a low dose of a second agent, such as nicotinic acid, gemfibrozil, or cholestyramine. Drugs from two different classes are sometimes necessary to achieve maximum therapeutic response.

Chapter 17

1. F   2. T   3. F   4. T   5. T   6. F
7. essential (or primary)
8. increases
9. increasing peripheral resistance (causing vasoconstriction)
10. relax or dilate; decreasing
11. angiotensin II; aldosterone
12. Reflex tachycardia
13. fight-or-flight
14. f   15. c   16. a   17. b   18. c   19. b
20. c   21. g   22. d   23. a   24. b   25. d
26. c   27. a   28. b   29. d   30. a   31. a
32. b   33. c   34. b   35. a   36. b   37. a
38. d   39. a   40. c   41. c   42. d   43. a

44. a. The nurse should try to convince Mr. H to stop smoking, because this is a major risk factor for hypertension. The elevated lipids may indicate a second risk factor, and the possibility of changes to dietary habits or antihyperlipidemic drug therapy may be considered. General stress or anxiety can contribute to hypertension, and relaxation methods or removal of stressors should be explored.

    b. The serious long-term consequences of unmanaged hypertension, including stroke and MI, should be explained to Mr. H.

    c. The prescriber will consider adding a second antihypertensive drug from a different drug class.

45. a. Orthostatic hypotension may be causing the dizziness. Explaining to Ms. F to sit on the side of the bed a few minutes before standing might solve this problem.

    b. Cardiac rhythm abnormalities are one sign of possible hyperkalemia. When switched to a potassium-sparing diuretic, such as spironolactone, Ms. F should not supplement her diet with excess potassium.

    c. It may not be necessary to change this patient's medication, because it seems to be keeping blood pressure within normal limits. Patient teaching may be all that is necessary to resolve Ms. F's complaints.

46. a. Metabolism decreases the effectiveness of most drugs. In this case, propranolol decreases drug metabolism; thus, more of the nicardipine should remain in the blood and its effects will be enhanced. In addition, propranolol is an antihypertensive. The combined effects of the two drugs may cause significant hypotension.

    b. Both of these drugs slow the heart rate and bradycardia is a possibility. The patient may feel tired and suffer from dizziness and fainting episodes.

    c. Because both drugs lower blood pressure, the dose of nicardipine should probably be lowered when propranolol is added.

Chapter 18

1. F   2. F   3. T   4. T   5. F
6. workload
7. greater
8. 60   9. c   10. e   11. d   12. a   13. f
14. f   15. c   16. a   17. c   18. e   19. b
20. d   21. a   22. c   23. d   24. b   25. a
26. b   27. c   28. a   29. d   30. b   31. a
32. c   33. b   34. d   35. c   36. a   37. d
38. d   39. a   40. c   41. b   42. d   43. a
44. a. Inotropic drugs affect the strength of myocardial contraction. Chronotropic drugs affect the heart rate.

    b. Cardiac glycosides and the phosphodiesterase inhibitors are examples of drug classes that produce positive inotropic effects. Drugs that stimulate beta$_1$-adrenergic receptors and anticholinergics cause a positive chronotropic response.

    c. In HF, the heart should eject more blood per contraction; thus, positive inotropic drugs are needed. Positive chronotropic drugs are useful in treating cardiac failure and cardiogenic shock.

45. a. Hydrochlorothiazide and lisinopril will lower blood pressure, thus reducing the workload on Mr. L's heart. Atorvastatin will help reduce blood cholesterol levels, which are associated with hypertension and heart disease.

    b. Mr. L should be encouraged to take his medications as prescribed. He needs to understand that HF is a progressive disorder. He should be advised to try alternative therapies in addition to his medications, not in place of them.

    c. Mr. L should be advised to continue his walks and develop a complete exercise and dietary program under the direction of the health care provider.

Chapter 19

1. F   2. T   3. F   4. F   5. T   6. T
7. potassium
8. supraventricular
9. a. SA node
   b. AV node
   c. Bundle of His
   d. bundle branches
   e. Purkinje fibers
   f. P wave
   g. QRS complex
   h. T wave
10. a   11. c   12. b   13. d   14. e   15. d
16. a   17. a   18. b   19. a   20. e   21. a
22. a   23. d   24. c   25. d   26. b   27. c
28. a   29. d   30. d   31. c   32. b   33. a
34. b   35. b   36. d   37. d   38. c   39. b
40. c   41. a   42. c   43. a   44. d   45. c
46. b
47. a. Lidocaine is given IV to terminate serious ventricular dysrhythmias. Aspirin is given as an anticoagulant to prevent additional clots from forming. Hydromorphone is given for the severe pain associated with MI.

    b. Beta blockers will slow the heart rate and worsen the patient's bradycardia.

    c. In high amounts, digoxin can cause dysrhythmias and bradycardia, two symptoms Ms. D is experiencing. Dysrhythmias are common complications following an MI.

48. a. Digoxin benefits patients with heart failure and certain types of atrial dysrhythmias.

    b. Acebutolol, propranolol, sotalol, and verapamil are also used for hypertension.

c. Propranolol and verapamil are also used for migraines.

d. Phenytoin is a widely used seizure medication that is also valuable for certain dysrhythmias.

Chapter 20

1. T   2. T   3. T   4. F   5. F

6. a. prothrombin activator

   b. thrombin

   c. fibrinogen

7. a. plasmin

   b. plasminogen activator

8. a	9. e	10. c	11. b	12. g	13. c
14. f	15. f	16. e	17. g	18. d	19. b
20. a	21. a	22. c	23. b	24. d	25. a
26. d	27. c	28. c	29. b	30. a	31. c
32. d	33. d	34. c	35. b	36. b	37. d
38. a	39. b	40. a	41. b	42. a	43. d
44. c					

45. a. Ms. S should use caution when engaged in activities that can cause bleeding, such as shaving, brushing teeth, trimming nails, and using kitchen knives. A soft toothbrush and an electric razor are safe choices. Contact activities, because of their high risk for injury, should be avoided.

   b. Ms. S should report unusual bruising or bleeding, such as nosebleeds, bleeding gums, black or red stool, heavy menstrual periods, or spitting up blood.

   c. Aspirin and other medications containing salicylates should never be taken. Acetaminophen or ibuprofen could be used for headaches.

46. a. Alcohol abuse is a major irritant for GI ulcers and might have contributed to the perforation. If Mr. P was taking warfarin, this could have led to prolonged bleeding.

   b. Chronic alcohol abuse leads to cirrhosis of the liver. Because several key blood clotting factors are synthesized by the liver, alcoholics often have prolonged bleeding times.

   c. Immediate IM administration of vitamin K_1 could help reverse the anticoagulant effects of warfarin. Administration of an antifibrinolytic, such as aminocaproic acid, might reduce excessive bleeding from the ulcer site.

Chapter 21

1. T   2. F   3. F   4. F   5. F   6. T

7. F   8. F

9. angina pectoris

10. plaque

11. organic nitrates

12. transdermal patch

13. coronary artery

14. anticoagulants/antiplatelets

15. thrombus (or clot); bleeding

16. removal of an existing clot; prevention of additional thrombi

17. d	18. c	19. a	20. b	21. a	22. b
23. c	24. a	25. b	26. c	27. a	28. d
29. c	30. b	31. a	32. a	33. d	34. b
35. c	36. c	37. a	38. d	39. a	40. d
41. d	42. b	43. b	44. a	45. c	46. d
47. c	48. c	49. c	50. d	51. b	52. d
53. b	54. b	55. a	56. c		

57. a. Mr. M has several obvious risk factors for stroke: obesity, hypertension, and tobacco use.

   b. Reteplase was given to dissolve the cerebral thrombosis, furosemide to lower blood pressure, and heparin to prevent further thrombi from forming. On discharge, hydrochlorothiazide and diltiazem were given to lower blood pressure and aspirin to prevent further strokes.

   c. Mr. M suffered from a thrombotic stroke. If he had been given heparin after a hemorrhagic stroke, it would have prolonged the bleeding and worsened the stroke.

58. a. The isosorbide dinitrate is to prevent angina attacks and heart failure, the nitroglycerin to terminate angina attacks, the lisinopril for hypertension and heart failure.

   b. Ms. R needs to be urged to follow a medically supervised diet and exercise program. She also needs to cease tobacco use.

   c. Ms. R may have become tolerant to the effects of the organic nitrates. Her doses of these agents may need adjustment or she may need to be switched to other medications for a period of time. If her doses are already at the high range, her coronary occlusion(s) may be worsening and surgery may be indicated.

Chapter 22

1. T   2. F   3. T

4. circulatory

5. basic life support

6. sympathetic

7. alpha

8. crystalloids or fluid replacement agents

9. immune

10. foreign

11. reflex tachycardia

12. a	13. d	14. a	15. b	16. c	17. a
18. b	19. c	20. a	21. b	22. c	23. d
24. a	25. c	26. b	27. d	28. c	29. a
30. b	31. d	32. b	33. c	34. a	35. c
36. b	37. d	38. b	39. d	40. a	41. c
42. b					

43. a. Paramedics often have to make quick decisions on whom to treat first at an accident scene. Mr. V did not have life-threatening symptoms and other patients may have been more seriously injured.

b. In early shock, a patient may appear normal with average vital signs. As shock progresses, however, vital signs may quickly change.

c. Oxygen is given to ensure adequate oxygenation of the blood. Dextran is a colloid given IV to expand fluid volume. Norepinephrine is a potent vasoconstrictor used to reverse Mr. V's severe hypotension. Dobutamine will help the heart beat with more force, so that vital organs can receive blood and nutrients. Lidocaine is likely given to correct the dysrhythmia.

44. a. With the obvious head injury, neurogenic shock must be considered. The fact that Ms. F is comatose and has signs of neurologic damage supports this diagnosis.

b. Vasoconstrictors will likely be needed to maintain Ms. F's blood pressure and inotropic agents, such as dopamine (Intropin), may be useful in strengthening the force of myocardial contraction.

c. Because brain and/or spinal cord injury is possible, the neck and head should be immobilized. The patient must be continuously monitored, because basic life support may become necessary.

Chapter 23

1. F 2. F 3. T 4. F
5. distal
6. increase
7. a. efferent arteriole
   b. peritubular capillaries
   c. proximal tubule
   d. distal tubule
   e. collecting duct
   f. loop of Henle
   g. Bowman's capsule
   h. glomerulus
   i. afferent arteriole

8. a. 9. c 10. b 11. e 12. c 13. d
14. a 15. b 16. b 17. b 18. b 19. c
20. d 21. a 22. b 23. c 24. b 25. d
26. a 27. c 28. a 29. d 30. d 31. b
32. b 33. a 34. c 35. d 36. b 37. a
38. a 39. c 40. b 41. c 42. c 43. d
44. a 45. b 46. a

47. a. Verapamil is a calcium channel blocker given to Mr. S for his hypertension. Verapamil is also of value in treating angina and dysrhythmias. Hydrochlorothiazide, a thiazide diuretic, was also given for hypertension. Potassium chloride was given to prevent the development of hypokalemia caused by diuretic use.

b. Patients with hypertension need follow-up exams every few months to determine the effectiveness of

their medication and the progress of their disease. It is possible that Mr. S's dramatic lifestyle changes caused his blood pressure to return to normal levels. The symptoms he is experiencing are those of hyperkalemia and overuse of verapamil and hydrochlorothiazide.

c. Mr. S should be urged to have his blood pressure checked weekly, until a new baseline level is observed. The physician may want to discontinue the potassium supplements and one or both of the antihypertensive medications.

48. a. Ms. S is taking three drugs that irritate the stomach mucosa. It is not surprising that she is experiencing abdominal discomfort. Hydrocortisone and aspirin, if given in high enough doses, can cause bleeding, which may account for the blood in Ms. S's stools. In addition, an extremely low carbohydrate diet causes the body to burn fats for energy, creating ketoacids. Her CNS depression may be caused by an impending acidosis.

b. Ms. S needs to be placed on a less stringent diet plan. She should not be taking her husband's potassium supplement, unless directed to do so by her health care provider. Her hydrocortisone and aspirin should not be taken at the same time and should be taken with meals to avoid adverse GI effects. The physician may prescribe an H_2-receptor blocker or a proton-pump inhibitor to reduce the risk for peptic ulcers.

Chapter 24

1. T 2. F 3. T 4. F
5. Passive immunity
6. infections or cancer
7. rid the body of antigens
8. humoral
9. plasma; antibodies
10. immunosuppressants

11. b 12. a 13. c 14. a 15. d 16. c
17. a 18. c 19. a 20. c 21. a 22. a
23. d 24. c 25. c 26. b 27. c 28. d
29. a 30. c 31. c 32. d 33. a 34. b
35. c 36. a 37. d 38. a 39. c 40. a
41. a 42. c 43. d 44. a 45. b

46. a. Ampicillin is an antibiotic to fight the infection. Empirin with Codeine #2 is a drug combination containing the opioid codeine and aspirin that is effective for moderate pain. Ketoprofen is an NSAID that is used to suppress inflammation and will provide Mr. E with additional pain relief.

b. Glucocorticoids are extremely effective anti-inflammatory agents but are usually contraindicated when active infections are present, as is the case with Mr. E.

47. a. The process of inflammation is nonspecific and may be triggered by most foreign agents that enter the body. Inflammation is mediated by chemicals, such as histamine and prostaglandins. The immune response is

very specific to certain antigens and is mediated by lymphocytes. Some of these lymphocytes, in addition to their specific action, may secrete substances that also trigger the nonspecific inflammatory response.

b. All types of inflammation are treated by the same drug classes, regardless of the source of the inflammation. However, in order to dampen the immune response, immunosuppressants may be needed.

Chapter 25

1. F   2. T   3. F   4. T   5. F   6. T
7. F   8. F   9. T
10. Need from AU
11. mutations
12. nosocomial
13. superinfection
14. Penicillinase (or beta-lactamase)
15. cephalosporins
16. beta-lactamase inhibitor
17. aminoglycosides
18. a   19. f   20. b   21. e   22. e   23. d
24. c   25. b   26. a   27. g   28. f   29. b
30. d   31. g   32. f   33. h   34. e   35. c
36. a   37. c   38. c   39. d   40. b   41. c
42. d   43. c   44. d   45. d   46. d   47. b
48. b   49. b   50. a   51. d   52. a   53. a
54. c   55. b   56. d

57. The widespread use of antibiotics often leads to resistant strains. The longer the antibiotic is used, the larger will be the percentage of resistant strains. Therefore, it is likely that Ms. P will develop a problem referred to as acquired resistance. It is likely that the antibiotic will sooner or later become ineffective in treating her infection.

58. Sometimes, broad-spectrum antibiotics are prescribed until culture and sensitivity testing can be performed and the actual microbe can be identified. Once identified, specific drug therapy can be chosen, based on which antibiotic will be most effective.

Chapter 26

1. F   2. T   3. T   4. F   5. F   6. T
7. F
8. capsid; ribonucleic acid (RNA); deoxyribonucleic acid (DNA)
9. Antiretrovirals
10. rhinovirus
11. zidovudine (Retrovir, AZT)
12. neuraminidase inhibitors
13. amantadine (Symmetrel)
14. acyclovir (Zovirax)
15. metronidazole (Flagyl)

16. a   17. b   18. a   19. a   20. b   21. a
22. c   23. a   24. d   25. b   26. e   27. f
28. d   29. d   30. d   31. c   32. a   33. c
34. b   35. d   36. a   37. a   38. d   39. c
40. a   41. a   42. b   43. c   44. a   45. b
46. a   47. a   48. d

49. There are many different antifungal drugs used for the treatment of candidiasis, including creams, lotions, and oral and IV medications. Of foremost importance is treatment of the condition without causing harm to the unborn child. It is important that the antifungal drug have no serious adverse effects. Examples of antifungals used for general infections for which adverse effects should be considered include amphotericin B (Fungizone, others), fluconazole (Diflucan), ketoconazole (Nizoral), and flucytosine (Ancobon). Less adverse and more common antifungals used specifically for vaginal candidiasis are terconazole (Terazol) and tioconazole (Vagi stat). The patient should consult her obstetrician concerning the best choice of drug.

50. The standard treatment for HIV/AIDS involves treatment with several drugs at the same time, a regimen described in the text as highly active antiretroviral therapy (HAART). With this approach, it is thought that HIV can be reduced to its lowest possible level in the blood. Although this approach does not eradicate HIV, it allows the patient to live symptom free much longer.

Chapter 27

1. F   2. F   3. F   4. T   5. T   6. T
7. F   8. T   9. T
10. chemotherapy
11. surgery; radiation therapy; multiple drugs; special dosing schedules
12. liposomes
13. alkylating agents
14. methotrexate
15. intravenous
16. vinca alkaloids; taxoids; topoisomerase inhibitors
17. Biologic response modifiers
18. a   19. b   20. e   21. b   22. c   23. d
24. e   25. d   26. f   27. a   28. b   29. a
30. d   31. d   32. c   33. a   34. c   35. a
36. c   37. b   38. c   39. d   40. b   41. c
42. a   43. d   44. d   45. a   46. b   47. a
48. d   49. b

50. Tumors should be treated at an early stage with multiple drugs and using several methods, such as chemotherapy, radiation, and surgery, whenever possible. If Mr. U has not sought medical therapy early enough, remaining cancer cells could decrease the chance for recovery. In addition, drugs from

different antineoplastic classes could be given during a course of chemotherapy. Different classes might affect different stages of the cancer cells' life cycle, thereby increasing the percentage of cancer cell death. Another approach is to administer drugs with specific dosing schedules to give normal cells time to recover from the adverse effects of the drugs.

51. Nausea and vomiting may be treated with drugs such as antiemetics, benzodiazepines, serotonin receptor blockers, and corticosteroids. To lower the risk of infection, the patient should avoid crowds, unsanitary conditions, and other potentially infectious situations. Proper hygiene is strongly recommended. Anorexia can be reduced by providing the patient with her favorite foods. A well-balanced diet should be implemented, including consultation with a registered dietitian.

Chapter 28

1. F   2. T   3. T   4. T   5. F
6. nebulizers
7. antihistamines, glucocorticoids, mast cell stabilizers
8. antihistamines
9. sympathomimetics
10. b   11. d   12. a   13. c   14. c   15. b
16. d   17. a   18. b   19. a   20. d   21. a
22. a   23. a   24. c   25. b   26. d   27. c
28. a   29. a   30. b   31. a   32. d   33. c
34. b   35. d

36. a. Beclomethasone is a glucocorticoid that is taken to prevent asthmatic attacks, and propranolol is a nonselective beta blocker that was likely prescribed for hypertension.

b. The patient was taking the beclomethasone incorrectly. This drug is ineffective at terminating acute asthmatic attacks. As a beta blocker, propranolol causes bronchoconstriction and is usually contraindicated in patients with asthma. There are many safer choices of antihypertensives for patients with asthma.

c. Lorazepam is a benzodiazepine that was used to calm Mr. H in the ED. Metaproterenol activates beta$_2$-receptors and is used for bronchodilation to relieve Mr. H's severe shortness of breath.

37. a. Novahistine contains codeine (antitussive), pseudoephedrine (decongestant), and guaifenesin (expectorant). It is prescribed to relieve severe flu symptoms.

b. Acetaminophen is an antipyretic used to reduce fever. Aspirin use in children with fever is associated with a small risk for Reye's syndrome; therefore, acetaminophen is often the preferred drug.

Chapter 29

1. T   2. T   3. T   4. T   5. F
6. sphincter
7. simethicone

8. nausea; vomiting
9. anorexiants
10. a   11. a   12. i   13. b   14. c   15. j
16. a   17. h   18. b   19. h   20. e   21. d
22. d   23. d   24. a   25. c   26. c   27. b
28. a   29. d   30. a   31. c   32. d   33. d
34. a   35. b   36. a   37. d   38. c   39. a
40. b   41. b   42. d   43. a   44. c

45. a. The evening pain and vomiting are more characteristic of a gastric ulcer.

b. Alcohol and tobacco use contribute significantly to gastric acid production and peptic ulcer formation.

c. The antacids taken by Mr. D are ineffective at healing ulcers. Mr. D would likely improve on a regimen of antibiotics (to treat *H. pylori*) and an H$_2$-receptor blocker, such as ranitidine. Another option would be a proton-pump inhibitor, such as omeprazole (Prilosec).

46. a. Elderly patients sometimes become concerned about having daily bowel movements and resort to overuse of laxatives. Overuse can decrease the muscular tone of the colon muscles and lead to additional laxative use. As is the case with Ms. V, the frequency of bowel movements declines with low food intake and lack of exercise. Ms. V should be encouraged to add fiber to her diet in the form of fruits and vegetables and to start a medically supervised exercise program.

b. Phenolphthalein laxatives are stimulants that are not intended to be taken daily. A better choice for Ms. V is the bulk-forming natural laxatives, such as psyllium mucilloid. These add bulk to the stool, which encourages natural contractions of the bowel.

Chapter 30

1. F   2. T   3. T   4. F   5. F   6. T
7. T   8. K
9. iron deficiency anemia
10. fat
11. recycled through the liver
12. a   13. a   14. b   15. b   16. b   17. b
18. d   19. a   20. a   21. c   22. d   23. b
24. a   25. c   26. a   27. d   28. c   29. d
30. a   31. b   32. b   33. c   34. b   35. c
36. b   37. d   38. a   39. a

40. a. The patient is fundamentally correct when he states that all necessary nutrients can be obtained through a normal diet. However, you must assess whether the patient's intake is really normal and contains a sufficient quality and quantity of nutrients. Patients' self-perceptions of a balanced diet are often not accurate.

b. You must assess the level of physical activity of the patient as well as obtain a current medical history. High physical activity or a history of GI, liver, or kidney disease may warrant supplementation.

c. Food intake often declines in elderly patients and absorption of nutrients is diminished. They are also more likely to have chronic diseases that place unusual nutritional demands on the body.

Chapter 31

1. F   2. F   3. F   4. T   5. T   6. T
7. F   8. T
9. Hormones
10. pituitary
11. electrolyte
12. IV
13. cardiovascular
14. anxiety
15. with
16. infection
17. type 1 diabetes mellitus; type 2 diabetes mellitus
18. oral hypoglycemics
19. resistant
20. blood glucose
21. severe epigastric pain
22. Alcohol
23. c   24. d   25. e   26. a   27. b   28. c
29. b   30. a   31. b   32. c   33. a   34. c
35. b   36. a   37. d   38. d   39. c   40. b
41. a   42. a   43. b   44. d   45. c   46. d
47. d   48. a   49. a   50. b   51. a   52. c
53. c   54. d   55. d   56. d   57. b   58. a
59. b   60. c   61. c   62. c   63. b   64. a
65. d   66. c   67. b   68. a   69. b   70. a
71. a. Thyroid preparations increase metabolic activity. They may elevate body temperature, increase heart rate, and reduce the patient's weight. The effects of thyroid medications increase when a patient is also taking insulin.

b. The nurse should take a thorough health history, communicate findings with the prescribing physician, and teach the patient to report adverse effects promptly.

72. a. PTU may cause vital sign changes. The patient should be taught how to monitor these and to report changes promptly. This may require the purchase of necessary equipment. Risk of infection increases with the use of PTU. The patient must understand the importance of avoiding crowds and individuals with known illnesses. This may lead to feelings of isolation.

b. The nurse can assist by encouraging alternative methods of communication, such as the telephone and computer, when susceptibility is increased. Because drowsiness may occur with the use of this medication, teaching concerning safety is of importance. The nurse should instruct the patient to avoid being near environmental hazards, driving, and operating machinery.

73. a. Pharmacotherapy for type 2 diabetes is usually oral hypoglycemic agents, and lifestyle changes, such as

proper diet and increased level of activity, will be necessary.

b. Because Mr. D is elderly, these approaches may be a problem, because older patients are not as active as the general population and they do not easily comply with instructions for a change of diet. Additionally, if Mr. D has other physical limitations because of his age or if he is not able to receive proper instruction because of these limitations (seeing or hearing, for example), these could be obstacles to diabetic therapy.

74. a. The nurse must communicate to Mr. C the importance of avoiding alcohol; cigarette smoking; and spicy, gas-forming foods. He should weigh himself daily; observe stools for color, frequency, and consistency changes; and eat a diet low in fat.

b. This patient needs fresh foods but, with a fixed income, may be unable to afford the foods that are best for him. The nurse may need to refer this patient to social services, which can connect him with agencies that may be able to provide meals and transportation.

75. a. Potassium iodide prevents damage to the thyroid gland *only* after radiation exposure. It *does not* protect any other tissues. It will not prevent radiation sickness or other cancers that may develop as a result of the exposure.

b. Potassium iodide will be absorbed by the thyroid gland and prevent the radioactive iodine from being absorbed by the gland. This lessens the gland's exposure to radiation and prevents the cancer. KI is effective if taken 3 to 4 hours after exposure.

Chapter 32

1. T   2. F   3. F   4. T   5. T   6. F
7. T   8. F   9. T   10. F   11. F   12. T
13. T   14. F
15. Follicle-stimulating hormone; luteinizing hormone
16. menopause
17. conjugated estrogens
18. amenorrhea
19. progestins
20. prolactin; oxytocin
21. Anabolic steroids
22. virulization
23. sildenafil (Viagra)
24. Benign prostatic hyperplasia (BPH)
25. b   26. a   27. d   28. e   29. c   30. b
31. c   32. a   33. f   34. e   35. d   36. d
37. d   38. d   39. b   40. a   41. b   42. a
43. c   44. b   45. d   46. a   47. c   48. c
49. c   50. c   51. a   52. b   53. c   54. d
55. d   56. b
57. a. Ms. M has a knowledge deficit related to the prescribed drug regimen. The desired outcome is for

Ms. M to understand the drug regimen and manage her regimen appropriately.

b. Estrogen replacement therapy may be prescribed short-term to alleviate unpleasant symptoms occurring during and after menopause. Hot flashes, night sweats, vaginal dryness, susceptibility to infection, erratic menstrual cycle, and nervousness may be reduced. The short-term risks of estrogen replacement therapy are bloating, nausea, vaginal bleeding, breast tenderness, and other common menstrual symptoms. The long-term risks of estrogen replacement therapy are ovarian cancer, gallbladder disease, and breast cancer.

58. a. The nurse must use this medication with caution and continuously monitor maternal and fetus status. Adverse effects of oxytocin include fetal dysrhythmias, neonatal jaundice, and intracranial hemorrhage related to possible fetal trauma. Maternal effects include cardiac arrhythmias, hypertensive episodes, water intoxication, uterine rupture or uterine hypotonicity, seizures, postpartum hemorrhage, and coma.

b. Changes in maternal and fetal vital signs must be reported immediately and the infusion stopped. Intake and output should be monitored closely. Contraction status during labor and fundal checks in the postpartum period are of utmost importance. The nurse must understand that uterine hypotonicity in the postpartum period is related to postpartum hemorrhage.

59. a. The nurse should teach Mr. E that the goal of finasteride (Proscar) therapy is to reduce urinary symptoms related to an enlarged prostate. Urinary symptoms such as hesitancy, difficulty starting the stream, decreased diameter of the stream, nocturia, dribbling, and frequency should be diminished. The nurse should explain to Mr. E that is may be necessary to take Proscar for the remainder of his life to keep the symptoms under control.

b. To evaluate the effectiveness of the therapy, the nurse should devise a method of follow-up to assess the resolution of urinary symptoms. Mr. E should also be encouraged to contact his nurse if symptoms worsen.

60. a. The nurse should obtain a list of herbs used by Mr. S. If he uses echinacea in conjunction with androgen therapy, his insulin requirements may decrease, necessitating a change in his insulin dosage.

b. Mr. S should be instructed to monitor his blood glucose carefully during androgen therapy and be encouraged to report symptoms of hypoglycemia, such as sweating, anxiety, or vertigo.

Chapter 33

1. F   2. F   3. T   4. F   5. T   6. T

7. T

8. movement

9. nervous; muscular; endocrine; skeletal

10. calcium

11. parathyroid; thyroid

12. vitamin D

13. rickets

14. osteoporosis; Paget's disease

15. parathyroid hormone; calcitonin

16. calcifediol; calcitriol

17. complexed; elemental

18. Selective estrogen receptor modulators (SERMs)

19. bisphosphonates

20. bisphosphonates; calcitonin

21. Disease-modifying drugs

22. uric acid inhibitors

23. b   24. a   25. e   26. c   27. d   28. e
29. c   30. c   31. a   32. b   33. d   34. e
35. c   36. b   37. d   38. d   39. a   40. c
41. b   42. b   43. d   44. b   45. c   46. a
47. d   48. c   49. a   50. d   51. b   52. b
53. b   54. a   55. d   56. c   57. b   58. a

59. a. The symptoms the patient is experiencing are normal for his condition. Allopurinol (Lopurin) is used for gout flare-up and primary and secondary hyperuricemia.

b. To allay the pain, NSAIDs would probably be administered with antigout therapy. Medications could be administered with meals to minimize gastric upset. Other expected effects include diarrhea and rash. Precautions would be taken to minimize these symptoms. Over a longer time, difficulty in urination may occur.

c. During drug therapy, laboratory tests (BUN and creatinine) would be ordered to monitor whether the kidneys are functioning properly. Fluid intake and output would be monitored. Because allopurinol may cause bone marrow depression, blood cell counts would be taken regularly. Liver function tests would also be ordered.

60. a. Patients with kidney disease are unable to synthesize the active form of vitamin D from the precursors formed by the body or taken in the diet. Calcium is not absorbed well from the GI tract unless there is adequate vitamin D, so the patient may become hypocalcemic.

b. The patient should be informed that periodic liver function tests will be necessary as well as calcium, magnesium, and phosphate levels. The drug should be taken exactly as directed, so that toxic levels do not develop. Fatigue, weakness, nausea, and vomiting should be reported. Alcohol and other liver toxic drugs should be avoided. Exposure to 20 minutes of sunlight daily will help increase the amount of vitamin D available to the patient.

c. The importance of routine laboratory studies for calcium levels must be stressed. Oral calcium supplements should be taken with meals or within an hour after meals. The patient should be advised to consume calcium-rich foods, such as dark green, leafy vegetables and dairy products.

61. a. Osteoporosis occurs when the rate of bone replacement is less than the rate of bone breakdown. People at risk for osteoporosis include postmenopausal women; those who use excess alcohol or caffeine; those with anorexia nervosa; smokers; inactive persons; those who lack adequate vitamin D or calcium in their diets; and persons using corticosteroids, antiseizure medications, and immunosuppressive drugs. The disease can be detected through the use of bone density tests.

b. Medications used to treat osteoporosis include calcium and vitamin D therapy, estrogen replacement therapy, estrogen receptor modulators, bisphosphonates, and calcitonin.

c. The patient will need to be instructed that alendronate (Fosamax) decreases the breakdown of her bones. The usual side effects are GI problems, such as nausea, vomiting, abdominal pain, and esophageal irritation. The drug should be taken on an empty stomach once a week. To prevent the esophagus from becoming irritated, the patient should not lie down for 30 minutes after taking the medication. Patient teaching for raloxifene (Evista) should include the need for periodic bone density scans. Sudden chest pain, dyspnea, pain in the calves, and swelling in the legs should be reported promptly. The patient should not take estrogen replacement therapy while using this drug. In addition, safety measures regarding falls should be discussed as well as the need for weight-bearing activity and adequate dietary consumption of calcium and vitamin D.

Chapter 34

1. F	2. F	3. T	4. T	5. T	6. T
7. F	8. T	9. T			

10. keratolytic
11. scabies
12. retinoids
13. emollients
14. pruritus
15. antibiotics; oral contraceptives
16. eczema
17. papules

18. c	19. d	20. e	21. c	22. a	23. b
24. c	25. d	26. c	27. e	28. a	29. b
30. c	31. b	32. a	33. d	34. d	35. d
36. c	37. b	38. b	39. d	40. a	41. a
42. b	43. b	44. c	45. d	46. c	

47. a. Permethrin should be used cautiously in children under 10 years of age, and only if other pediculicides fail. Because this is the case here, the mother needs to know that some antiparasitic agents cause local skin irritation and adverse CNS effects, such as restlessness,

dizziness, tremors, or convulsions. This usually occurs after misuse or ingestion. Any shampoos or topical agents must be kept out of the reach of smaller children in the household. They should not be applied to open skin lesions or used if the child has seizures. The mother should wear gloves while applying shampoos, particularly if she is pregnant. Any scabicide should remain on the hair for at least 5 minutes. Use of tepid water will decrease itching.

b. The child's school nurse or teacher should be notified, as should the parents of the child with whom she spent the night and any other children who attended the sleepover. Anyone else with whom the child has had close contact (grandparents, for example) should be notified as well.

c. Children in school should not swap clothing or towels. Coat and hat racks at school may need to be eliminated to prevent the spread from one child to another. Combs or other hygiene supplies should not be shared, and bodily contact with an infected person should be avoided. Also, the child should not sleep with brothers or sisters until the problem is resolved. The nurse should stress that this is not a problem of social class but simply an event that occurs when there is close contact.

48. a. You would ask the patient if he has had nausea, vomiting, chills, and headache, as well as assess the amount of pain and extent of the erythema. Also ask about sunburn and tanning history, the amount of time the patient usually spends in the sun before beginning to burn, and if he uses sunscreen products. An allergy history is also necessary.

b. Soothing lotions, rest, prevention of dehydration, and topical anesthetic agents may help. The topical anesthetics may be chilled prior to application to increase the cooling effect. In severe cases, aspirin or ibuprofen may be used.

c. Medication should not be applied to broken skin. If this occurs, call the doctor. Prevent sunburn by decreasing exposure to sunlight or by increasing the SPF number of the sunscreen. Wear a broad-brimmed hat, UV protection for the eyes, and a long-sleeved shirt if extended exposure to sunlight is expected during peak hours of the day. Sunburn results from overexposure to UV light and is associated with light skin complexions. Chronic sun exposure can lead to eye injury, cataracts, and skin cancer.

49. a. Causes of acne are unknown, although some factors associated with it have been identified. Overproduction of sebum by oil glands, keratin that blocks oil glands, and certain bacteria grow within oil gland openings and change the sebum to an irritating substance. This results in small, inflamed bumps on the skin. Other factors include male hormones, which regulate the activity of the sebaceous glands.

b. A mental health history should be taken to determine whether the patient has a history of depression or suicidal tendencies. Patients with seizures who use carbamazepine should be identified, because there is an increased risk for seizures. Also, oral antidiabetic agents may not be as effective, so you should assess for diabetes, heart disease, and elevated lipid levels. Prior to using the drug, a patch test must be done to test for sensitivity.

c. He should be told to monitor foods and avoid those that seem to make his acne worse. He can be taught to keep a food log to help determine which ones these are. Products that will irritate the skin, such as cologne, perfumes, and other alcohol-based products, should be avoided. If severe inflammation occurs during therapy, the physician should be notified. Use of OTC agents should be avoided unless approved by the physician.

Chapter 35

1. T   2. F   3. T   4. F   5. T   6. T
7. T
8. blockage; outflow
9. open-angle glaucoma
10. miotics
11. mydriatics
12. cycloplegics
13. external otitis
14. otitis media
15. mastoiditis
16. cerumen
17. a   18. b   19. b   20. b   21. a   22. a
23. a   24. g   25. h   26. c   27. b   28. d
29. e   30. f   31. b   32. b   33. b   34. a
35. c   36. d   37. d   38. c   39. a   40. b
41. a   42. c   43. a   44. a   45. d   46. b
47. b   48. a   49. a   50. a

51. These is no need to verify the order—this is the standard way to administer pilocarpine in an emergency situation. (Of course, if you are unsure of anything, it is always best to check it out before you go ahead.)

52. a. There is no permanent cure for glaucoma. Medications will have to be used indefinitely. Several classes of eye medications may be used alone or in combination to control the intraocular pressure problem characteristic of glaucoma.

b. Xalatan is used to decrease the IOP. Side effects may include conjunctival edema, tearing, dryness, burning, pain, itching, photophobia, or visual disturbances. The eyelashes on the treated eye may grow, thicken, and darken. The iris may have

color changes, as well as the skin around the eye. Generalized flulike symptoms may occur. The patient should remove contacts prior to administering, leave them out for 15 minutes, and wait 5 minutes between different eye medications.

c. The patient should be instructed to report any visual changes and any changes in medications or new health-related problems. He should be taught the proper way to administer eyedrops and told to schedule them around his daily routines. Signs of side effects should be reported. He will need to know that measurements of intraocular pressure will be done periodically. For his safety, environmental lighting needs to be adjusted when it is dark and may need to be dimmed if there is photophobia.

d. Intraocular pressure should be measured using tonometry at regular intervals to determine the effectiveness of the medication.

53. a. Additional assessments needed include Timmy's allergy history and whether his mother knows how to administer the drugs properly and is aware of potential side effects.

b. Mrs. B needs teaching regarding the correct use of eardrops and the fact that aspirin is contraindicated in young children due to the risk for Reye's syndrome. Teaching should include the following: Eardrops are contraindicated in cases where the eardrum has perforated. This is the most likely cause of the drainage in Timmy's ear, and it may be seen on examination of the tympanic membrane. Explain that the bacteria present in the outer ear may be carried into the middle ear when the drops run in, thus increasing the chances for a further infection. Timmy's mother needs to be made aware that eardrops should be warmed by holding the container under warm water prior to administration. Also, the child should lie on the side opposite the affected ear for 5 minutes after the drops are put in. If the child is older than 3 years, the pinna should be pulled up and back; if younger than 3 years, it should be pulled down and back.

54. a. Mrs. I probably has impacted cerumen (earwax). This would explain the mild hearing loss and a sensation of fullness with intermittent ringing of the ears. Other assessments to make would include whether she has a history of ruptured tympanic membranes, auditory canal surgery, or myringotomy tubes, because these would contraindicate an ear irrigation and the use of earwax softeners.

b. Initial nursing interventions would include removal by using mineral oil or an earwax softener preparation followed by irrigation with a bulb syringe.